Library of Congress Cataloging-in-Publication Data

ISBN: 978-1-53617-286-7

Published by Nova Science Publishers, Inc. † New York

CONTENTS

PREFACE

Before the ACA, sick people often couldn't get health insurance due to a pre-existing condition. If they were able to get coverage, they often paid significantly more for it than someone without a pre-existing condition. Today, millions of Americans no longer have to worry about large bills due to annual or lifetime limits on benefits. Yet, there is still a serious affordability problem in the individual market, especially for those who rely on the individual market for coverage but are not eligible for financial assistance and those facing rising deductibles. Chapters 1 discuss ways to stabilize premiums and help individuals obtain affordable insurance through the individual insurance market.

Healthcare reform should empower individuals and families to make decisions for themselves based on what fits their needs and their budget. One of the best tools we have to accomplish this goal is consumer-directed health plans that are paired with health savings accounts, or HSAs. These plans offer lower premiums and a higher deductible to encourage better use of healthcare services as examined in chapter 2.

IHS provides care to American Indians and Alaska Natives through a system of health care facilities. The Patient Protection and Affordable Care Act (PPACA) provided states with the option to expand their Medicaid programs, and created new coverage options beginning in 2014, including for American Indians and Alaska Natives. Chapter 3 describes (1) trends in health insurance coverage and third-party collections at federally operated and tribally operated facilities from fiscal years 2013 through 2018, and (2) the effects of any changes in coverage and collections on these facilities.

Chapter 1 - This is an edited, reformatted and augmented version of Testimony before the United States Senate Committee on Health, Education, Labor, and Pensions, dated September 6, 2017.

Chapter 2 - This is an edited, reformatted and augmented version of Hearing before the Subcommittee on Health, of the Committee on Ways and Means, U.S. House of Representatives, One Hundred Fifteenth Congress, Second Session, Serial No. 115-HL07, dated June 6, 2018.

Chapter 3 - IHS provides care to American Indians and Alaska Natives through a system of health care facilities. The Patient Protection and Affordable Care Act (PPACA) provided states with the option to expand their Medicaid programs, and created new coverage options beginning in 2014, including for American Indians and Alaska Natives. GAO was asked to review how PPACA has affected health care coverage and services for American Indians and Alaska Natives. In this chapter, GAO describes (1) trends in health insurance coverage and third-party collections at federally operated and tribally operated facilities from fiscal years 2013 through 2018, and (2) the effects of any changes in coverage and collections on these facilities. To address these objectives, GAO analyzed IHS data on coverage, third-party collections, and PRC. GAO interviewed IHS officials from headquarters and all 12 area offices, as well as from 17 facilities selected to include a mix of federally operated and tribally operated hospitals and health centers in states that both had and had not expanded their Medicaid programs as of September 2018. GAO interviewed officials from 11 federally operated IHS facilities and 6 tribally operated facilities. GAO provided a draft of this chapter to the Secretary of Health and Human Services for comment. The Department did not have any comments on the draft report.

In: Health Insurance
Editor: Cory Oliver
ISBN: 978-1-53617-286-7

Chapter 1

STABILIZING PREMIUMS AND HELPING INDIVIDUALS IN THE INDIVIDUAL INSURANCE MARKET FOR 2018: STATE INSURANCE COMMISSIONERS*

Teresa Miller

Good morning Chairman Alexander, Ranking Member Murray, and members of the U.S. Senate Committee on Health, Education, Labor, and Pensions. Thank you for the opportunity to be here today to speak about an issue that is so critical for residents of the Commonwealth of Pennsylvania.

I am pleased to have been recently chosen by Governor Wolf to serve as acting secretary for the Pennsylvania Department of Human Services after having been Insurance Commissioner since shortly after Gov. Wolf took office in 2015.

Gov. Wolf has been an active participant in a group of governors working to ensure Congress's approach to health care reform is completed

---

* This is an edited, reformatted and augmented version of Testimony before the United States Senate Committee on Health, Education, Labor, and Pensions, dated September 6, 2017.

in a bi-partisan manner that strengthens our nation's health insurance system. Additionally, the governors urge Congress to takes steps to make coverage more affordable and stable in the interim.

Both Gov. Wolf and I applaud the committee's efforts to work towards a solution on this important issue. As we begin to talk about the importance of stabilizing our individual health insurance markets under the Affordable Care Act (ACA), we should first recognize the impact that the ACA itself has had on Pennsylvanians and why it is imperative that we fix the law rather than undoing the progress we have made. Before the ACA, sick people often couldn't get health insurance due to a pre-existing condition. If they were able to get coverage, they often paid significantly more for it than someone without a pre-existing condition. In some cases, these individuals would be offered a policy, but it would not include coverage for their pre-existing condition. Individuals with chronic medical issues or anyone who underwent a costly procedure like a transplant could face financially devastating annual and lifetime limits. Women could see higher monthly premiums than men and perhaps not have contraception or maternity care covered. Other critical services like mental health and substance use disorder treatment services and prescription drugs were often difficult if not impossible to find coverage for. Most importantly, more than 10 percent of Pennsylvanians and 16 percent of Americans nationwide went uninsured.

Since the ACA's passage, the national uninsured rate has fallen to 8.6 percent and Pennsylvania's uninsured rate has dropped to 6.4 percent – the lowest it's ever been. More than 1.1 million Pennsylvanians have accessed coverage through the ACA, and that coverage is much more comprehensive than what was previously available. There are 12.7 million Pennsylvanians, and more than 40 percent of them – 5.4 million – have pre-existing conditions and cannot be denied health insurance coverage due to the ACA. Today, 4.5 million Pennsylvanians no longer have to worry about large bills due to annual or lifetime limits on benefits, and 6.1 million Pennsylvanians benefit from access to free preventive care services. In addition to this, more than 175,000 Pennsylvanians have also been able to access substance use disorder treatment services through their exchange and Medicaid expansion coverage. These services are critical as our commonwealth and other states around the country strive to combat the overwhelming impact of the opioid epidemic.

The positive impact of the governor's efforts to expand Medicaid and help Pennsylvanians access treatment services for substance use disorder have become even more evident to me as I've taken the helm at the Department of Human Services. These are expansions that are making a significant difference in people's lives.

While the ACA has not been perfect, it is critical that we level set and talk about the issues that exist and who those issues really impact. The ACA has had minimal impact on the Medicare program and enhanced the already very popular Medicaid program by expanding access to millions more around the country. Further, since the passage of the ACA, the employer markets, where small and large businesses can purchase insurance products for their employees, have been stable and even seen costs grow at a slower pace than before the ACA. The individual market, where we see problems, is a very small market relative to these others, covering only about 5 percent of Pennsylvanians. However, this market is very important because it is where individuals and families who do not have access to coverage through their employer or public programs go to purchase insurance.

This market is heavily subsidized because of the ACA. About 80 percent of Pennsylvanians who purchase their coverage through the exchange receive tax credits to help pay their premiums. Because of the way the tax credits are structured based on income, these consumers do not feel the full impact of premium increases. Currently more than half of Pennsylvania consumers who enroll in the exchanges are also eligible for cost-sharing reductions, additional financial assistance that helps them pay for their out-of-pocket costs like deductibles and co-pays. The payments the federal government makes to insurers to cover the costs of this additional financial assistance are in jeopardy because President Trump has not committed to making them longer than a month-to-month basis. I am seriously concerned about the destabilizing effect failing to commit to these payments could have on both Pennsylvania's market and others around the country and how this will impact premiums for people in the individual market, but I will address this at length later in this testimony.

I believe we need to build upon the foundation of the health care system we have and make targeted, common sense changes that will improve the ACA and make it work better for the people it is not working perfectly for today. We still have a serious affordability problem in the individual market, especially for the 1-2 percent of Pennsylvanians who rely on the individual market for coverage but are not eligible for financial assistance and those facing rising deductibles. Their concerns are legitimate and must be addressed, but starting over or moving backwards will not better serve Pennsylvanians or Americans throughout the nation. I applaud this committee's efforts to work together to strengthen this law so it may better serve everyone rather than undoing the good it has accomplished around the country. With that context, I would like to offer Pennsylvania's thoughts on the issues we currently face and what reasonable bipartisan solutions that would improve the ACA for all could look like.

Guaranteeing Payments for Cost-Sharing Reductions

While the individual market is facing issues, in some states more than in others, I can tell you that Pennsylvania's market is on a path to stability and will not implode unless the federal government takes adverse action. Our market saw some issues last year and lost two carriers, but I worked closely with our remaining insurers to ensure that we did not have any bare counties for 2017. For 2018, our individual market insurers filed for a statewide average increase of just 8.8 percent, assuming no changes come from the federal level. An analysis on the drivers of 2018 premium increases puts our requests at or below what we would expect based on trends in annual medical costs and a federal tax on health insurance plans that comes into effect for the 2018 plan year. I am very happy that our insurers are finally seeing improved experience with this market and that is reflected in the rate increases they filed, but I am very concerned that this stability is on fragile ground because of all the uncertainty here in Washington.

When rates were initially filed, I asked our insurers to provide information on what they would need to request if cost-sharing reduction payments were not made or if the individual mandate was not enforced. The differences are stark. If cost-sharing reductions are not paid, they estimated that they would need to request a statewide average increase of 20.3 percent. If the individual mandate is not enforced, they said they would seek an estimated 23.3 percent increase. If both changes occur, our insurers estimated that they would seek an estimated increase of 36.3 percent, assuming they continue to participate in the market at all. I'd be lying if I said these numbers didn't worry me, especially as we prepare to finalize rates. At this point, we have no more certainty on cost-sharing reductions than we had in April when I, along with executives from all five of Pennsylvania's on-exchange insurers, first wrote to Secretary Tom Price on this issue.

What's most frustrating about the situation we are in is that it is entirely avoidable. I have sent multiple letters to Secretary Price asking the administration to not take steps to undermine the progress we have made and the pathway to stability that we put our market on. I reiterated this urgent need for stability in an answer to a request for information on how to stabilize the individual market issued by the Centers for Medicare and Medicaid Services in June. Governor Wolf and a bi-partisan group of governors have asked Congressional leaders to address stability, too. And, yet here we are, two weeks out from when states need to send final rates for 2018 to the Department of Health and Human Services (HHS) – a deadline that was already extended – and the Trump Administration still refuses to make anything longer than a month-to-month commitment on these payments.

I cannot stress enough how difficult this uncertainty is on our insurers. These payments have a significant impact on their rates, and failing to make a long-term commitment will do nothing but drive up prices for consumers in the individual market. This will further hurt the 1 to 2 percent of Pennsylvanians – roughly 125,000 people – who do not receive subsidies as those who do receive subsidies would be shielded from most of the increases – if their insurer stayed in the market at all. At the end of the day, rates have to be finalized based on finite assumptions and insurers will sign contracts to participate on the exchange or they won't participate at all. Pennsylvania consumers will be left to bear the burden of premium increases or lessened choices necessitated by this instability.

Failing to make payments for cost-sharing reductions does not serve any goal aside from trying to make markets fail. According to the Congressional Budget Office's analysis on the matter, doing so would result in higher premiums, more counties without individual market coverage options for 2018, and would increase the federal deficit by $194 billion through 2026 due to the payment of additional premium subsidies because of higher premiums. The Congressional Budget Office further estimates that premiums would rise an additional 20 percent in 2018. This will undoubtedly create more problems, especially for individual market consumers who are not eligible for financial assistance.

If the Trump Administration is not going to do the right thing for consumers and stabilize the law, Congress should allocate funds to ensure payments for cost-sharing reductions continue for 2018. Making these payments is the simplest way to "fix" the ACA that I can offer. I fear that it will very soon be too late to avoid rate increases for 2018, so Congress must act quickly.

SUPPORTING OPPORTUNITIES FOR STATE INNOVATION

Under Section 1332 of ACA, states have the opportunity to obtain waivers on portions of the law as long as they do not increase the federal deficit, reduce affordability or quality of coverage sold in the state, or have a negative quantitative impact on the state's insured population. States currently must offer a public notice and comment period, hold public hearings, and pass legislation outlining the state's intent to pursue and implement a Section 1332 waiver. Governor Wolf and I join the sentiments outlined in the bipartisan plan presented by Governors Hickenlooper and Kasich to streamline the waiver process in order to improve state flexibility.

Changes that permit states to easily build upon waivers obtained and successfully implemented by other states, coordinating the waiver submission and approval process, and easing the process of applying for waiver extensions would be viewed favorably. We would value the ability to pursue a waiver without requiring action from our state's legislature. If states are making small, targeted changes to stabilize the market like what is needed now, the current process can be too long and cumbersome when you consider a state's budget cycle and legislative process. An extensive process should be in place if states were to make significant changes to the structure of their market, but streamlining the current process would allow states to use Section 1332 waivers to make incremental changes as issues arise. The Wolf Administration would also look favorably on the opportunity to combine multiple waivers into a coordinated effort and consider deficit neutrality across the comprehensive plan.

However, we strongly believe that the baseline coverage improvements that must be maintained during the waiver process must be preserved. Eliminating these provisions – often called "guardrails" would likely result in a race to the bottom. Insurance companies would sell plans that offer less comprehensive coverage at a lower monthly cost, leaving consumers vulnerable to large out-of-pocket costs when care is accessed – something we all do at some point. These protections exist to ensure that Americans around the country have access to equitable, quality coverage regardless of the state in which they reside. The baseline protections contained in the ACA and the coverage improvements that have resulted should not be jeopardized as we consider opportunities for greater state flexibility.

Preserving the Individual Mandate

Since the ACA was passed, the individual mandate has historically been an unpopular feature of the law. However, it is imperative to making sure the law functions as it was intended.

The ACA included a "three-legged stool" – the individual mandate, non-discrimination requirements for people with pre-existing conditions, and subsidies and cost-sharing reductions – that helps insurers balance the added risk of individuals with pre-existing conditions while avoiding the risk of adverse selection where people only enter the market when they are sick and need care. Proposals to replace the ACA have eliminated the mandate in exchange for a continuous coverage requirement. Because purchasing insurance would no longer be mandatory under a continuous coverage requirement, the people who seek coverage during the open enrollment period will likely be a less healthy population and the risk pool would deteriorate, thus driving up premiums for those who need coverage the most.

I know that the individual mandate is not popular, but we must have adequate incentives to encourage people to purchase coverage and bring healthy people into the market. Over time, this should help stabilize and even lower premiums for everyone as more young and healthy people enter the market and help offset the cost of sicker enrollees.

Adequate Funding for Risk Stabilization Programs

When the ACA was passed, it contained three premium stabilization programs to help insurers experiencing higher than anticipated claims as they adjusted to the new market. Two of these programs – risk corridors and reinsurance – were designed to be temporary and have expired, but many insurers around the country, including those in Pennsylvania, are still owed significant risk corridor payments. Last year, Highmark, one of the

Pennsylvania insurers, sued HHS for these payments, and the Pennsylvania Insurance Department filed an amicus brief in support of their suit because insurance companies who entered this market under a set of expectations should be made whole for payments they were anticipating. Many of these insurers experienced significant losses in the first few years, and making these payments would be a good way for the federal government to demonstrate good faith and a long-term commitment to the success of this market.

Both ACA replacement proposals considered by the U.S. House and Senate contained reinsurance programs for 2018. Implementing a reinsurance program would be another effective way to demonstrate a long-term commitment to the health of this market for insurers and consumers who rely on this market for coverage.

A $15 billion reinsurance program in the context of a careful, bipartisan approach to improving our health care system would be something I would view favorably, especially if the individual mandate were preserved and outreach was boosted to improve enrollment in individual market plans. The ACA's reinsurance program successfully moderated premiums while it was in place and the reintroduction of a long-term reinsurance program could be an effective way to scale back the premiums we currently see. Increasing participation in the individual market would create a more stable, healthy risk pool, while the reinsurance program would help off-set the costs of enrollees with abnormally high claims costs. Together, these steps would moderate premiums for all while retaining the critical protections and robust benefits required by the ACA.

CONTINUING ENROLLMENT OUTREACH PROGRAMS

Encouraging people to enroll in this market through active outreach programs is extremely important to ensuring the market's success. The health of any insurance market depends on the strength of its risk pool, and reduced enrollment strains the risk pool and contributes to rising costs for those in it. I worry about some steps the Trump Administration has taken that could further erode the risk pool, such as shortening the open enrollment period and ending HHS's contracts to support outreach and enrollment efforts for the marketplace. In total, the Trump Administration intends to spend $10 million nationwide on advertising for 2018 open enrollment compared to $100 million spent last year. The administration also recently announced that funding granted to health insurance navigator organizations to help people enroll was almost halved from levels given under the previous administration. I worry that these decisions will result in fewer people enrolling and relatively fewer healthy people enrolling, exacerbating the issues that already exist in the risk pool.

Pennsylvanians are accustomed to having three months to enroll in coverage. In the past, December 15 has been an important deadline because it was previously the last day to enroll in coverage that was effective January 1, but enrollment still continued for the remaining six weeks of open enrollment. During 2017 open enrollment, more than 130,000 Pennsylvanians enrolled in coverage after the initial December 15 deadline. That is roughly one third of our market. I am extremely concerned that a shortened open enrollment period coupled with low outreach from the federal government will catch consumers off guard and result in people who want or need coverage being left out of the market because they missed the enrollment window.

In Pennsylvania, we are working to ensure that our marketplace population and potential enrollees understand this change through our own insurance outreach program. We are working alongside insurers, health care providers, consumer advocates, and other stakeholders to reach our common goal of increasing covered Pennsylvanians and informing them of important changes to this year's open enrollment period. Encouraging enrollment helps everyone – people have access to coverage, insurers have a more robust risk pool, and providers are more likely to receive compensation for care provided. Overtime, a more robust risk pool should result in lower premiums for consumers. I hope the Trump Administration ultimately sees the value in this outreach too, but for now Pennsylvania will work to fill the gap created by the Administration.

ADDRESSING UNDERLYING COSTS OF HEALTH CARE

Stabilizing the individual market is an important first step to addressing cost concerns we hear from consumers, but we still need to get to the root of what really drives insurance costs: the cost of health care. To put it simply, insurance is expensive because the health care it pays for is expensive. Unfortunately, it gets more and more expensive every year, which means premiums will continue to rise every year even if there are no detrimental changes to the market.

We need to have a serious national conversation about how we can moderate the unsustainable growth in health care costs, especially in areas experiencing astronomical growth in cost like we currently see with pharmaceutical costs. There is no silver bullet to reduce the cost of health care and the conversation is not easy, but it is essential as we look to the future and the long-term viability of our health care system. We continue to look for solutions to these problems at the state level, but these are national problems that I believe merit national solutions. So, I am hoping all of you and your colleagues in Congress will work alongside the states in tackling this complex and multifaceted issue.

THE NEED FOR BI-PARTISANSHIP

While the health reform debate has without question been partisan, the goals we are trying to achieve are not, and recognizing the real problems that exist in our health care system should not be either. I am very thankful that we are finally moving in the direction of working together, and I am optimistic that the ideas shared today will be a strong foundation moving forward. We all want Americans to have access to the care they need and be able to afford that care. We also want them to have choices, and that means supporting a competitive health insurance marketplace that can provide that choice. Let's start by recognizing where consumers may not have that access or affordability, and let's understand where we are not supporting the competitive market we need. Then, taking a lead from Governor Wolf and the group of bipartisan governors, let's look for solutions that can solve those problems, both in the short-term and in the long-term.

As my testimony outlines, I believe some of those short-term strategies must be to provide clarity and stability of the rules in the market by appropriating funds to ensure payment of cost-sharing reductions and robustly enforcing the individual mandate while enhancing outreach and enrollment efforts to get more healthy people into the market and improve the risk pool. A reinsurance program could also contribute to stability and the moderation of premiums and show insurers that the government wants to work with them for the benefit of consumers – your constituents – to make this market an attractive place to do business. In the long-term, it is imperative that we begin to look for ways to moderate the growth of health care costs to ensure our health care system is sustainable and will meet the needs of those that need it now as well as those that will need to rely on it in the future. I am hopeful that we can move away from drastic proposals that would jeopardize the health and financial security of millions of Americans, and focus on solving real problems with common sense solutions like these.

Again, thank you for allowing me to speak with you today. I would be happy to take any questions that you might have.

In: Health Insurance
Editor: Cory Oliver
ISBN: 978-1-53617-286-7

Chapter 2

LOWERING COSTS AND EXPANDING ACCESS TO HEALTH CARE THROUGH CONSUMER-DIRECTED HEALTH PLANS*

Subcommittee on Human Resources

WITNESSES

Roy Ramthun
President and Founder, HSA Consulting Services, LLC
Witness Statement

Matt Eyles
President & CEO, America's Health Insurance Plans (AHIP)
Witness Statement

* This is an edited, reformatted and augmented version of Hearing before the Subcommittee on Health, of the Committee on Ways and Means, U.S. House of Representatives, One Hundred Fifteenth Congress, Second Session, Serial No. 115-HL07, dated June 6, 2018.

Jody Dietel
Chief Compliance Officer, WageWorks, Inc.
Witness Statement

Sherry Glied
Dean, New York University, Robert F. Wagner Graduate School of Public Service
Witness Statement

CHAIRMAN ROSKAM ANNOUNCES HEARING ON LOWERING COSTS AND EXPANDING ACCESS TO HEALTH CARE THROUGH CONSUMER-DIRECTED HEALTH PLANS

House Ways and Means Health Subcommittee Chairman Peter Roskam (R-IL) announced today that the Subcommittee will hold a hearing on "Lowering Costs and Expanding Access to Health Care through Consumer-Directed Health Plans." The hearing will examine trends in enrollment and demographics for health spending account holders and the benefits of consumer-directed health care. It will also examine policies designed to give more consumers access to tax-favored savings accounts, including Health Savings Accounts. The hearing will take place on Wednesday, June 6, 2018 in 1100 Longworth House Office Building, beginning at 11:00 AM.

In view of the limited time to hear witnesses, oral testimony at this hearing will be from invited witnesses only. However, any individual or organization may submit a written statement for consideration by the Committee and for inclusion in the printed record of the hearing.

Details for Submission of Written Comments

Please Note: Any person(s) and/or organization(s) wishing to submit written comments for the hearing record must follow the appropriate link on the hearing page of the Committee website and complete the informational forms. From the Committee homepage, http://waysandmeans.house.gov, select "Hearings." Select the hearing for which you would like to make a submission, and click on the link entitled, "Click here to provide a submission for the record." Once you have followed the online instructions, submit all requested information. ATTACH your submission as a Word document, in compliance with the formatting requirements listed below, by the close of business on Wednesday, June 20, 2018.

Formatting Requirements

The Committee relies on electronic submissions for printing the official hearing record. As always, submissions will be included in the record according to the discretion of the Committee. The Committee will not alter the content of your submission, but we reserve the right to format it according to our guidelines. Any submission provided to the Committee by a witness, any materials submitted for the printed record, and any written comments in response to a request for written comments must conform to the guidelines listed below. Any submission not in compliance with these guidelines will not be printed but will be maintained in the Committee files for review and use by the Committee.

All submissions and supplementary materials must be submitted in a single document via email, provided in Word format and must not exceed a total of 10 pages. Witnesses and submitters are advised that the Committee relies on electronic submissions for printing the official hearing record.

All submissions must include a list of all clients, persons and/or organizations on whose behalf the witness appears. The name, company, address, telephone, and fax numbers of each witness must be included in the body of the email. Please exclude any personal identifiable information in the attached submission.

Failure to follow the formatting requirements may result in the exclusion of a submission. All submissions for the record are final.

The Committee seeks to make its facilities accessible to persons with disabilities. Questions with regard to special accommodation needs in general (including availability of Committee materials in alternative formats) may be directed to the Committee as noted above. Note: All Committee advisories and news releases are available at

http://www.waysandmeans.house.gov/

LOWERING COSTS AND EXPANDING ACCESS TO HEALTHCARE THROUGH CONSUMER-DIRECTED HEALTH PLANS

Wednesday, June 6, 2018

House of Representatives, Subcommittee on Health, Committee on Ways and Means, Washington, D.C.

The subcommittee met, pursuant to call, at 11:01 a.m., in Room 1100, Longworth House Office Building, Hon. Peter J. Roskam [chairman of the subcommittee] presiding.

Chairman Roskam. The subcommittee will come to order.

Welcome to the Ways and Means Health Subcommittee hearing on lowering costs and expanding access to healthcare through consumer-directed health plans. It is my pleasure to welcome our four witnesses today as we continue our discussion on lowering healthcare costs and increasing access to affordable insurance options.

Healthcare reform should empower individuals and families to make decisions for themselves based on what fits their needs and their budget.

One of the best tools we have to accomplish this goal is consumer-directed health plans that are paired with health savings accounts, or HSAs. These plans offer lower premiums and a higher deductible to encourage better use of healthcare services.

Engaging consumers in their healthcare spending is critical to reining in our system's ever-increasing costs. These plans continue to increase in popularity, now covering more than 21.8 million Americans.

Today our panel will update us on how health savings accounts are working for American families and employers. We are going to hear interesting data on current enrollment trends and demographic information on millions of people enrolled in HSAs and other tax-preferred savings accounts. We will also discuss many benefits of consumer-directed health plans and their potential cost to lower overall costs.

I am also pleased to hear what role these plans can play in fostering more price transparency, something that we all have been discussing for quite some time. In addition, our witnesses will tell us about the barriers employers and individuals face when trying to offer or enroll in an HSA qualified plan. And, finally, we will examine the various reform ideas, including many authored by members of this subcommittee, that are aimed at expanding access to HSAs.

Our goal is to use this hearing as an opportunity to discuss how we can give more people this affordable option for coverage while still preserving the right structural incentives to bend the cost curve and keep premiums low.

I appreciate the knowledgeable testimonies of the witnesses here today, and this subcommittee looks forward to hearing comments, criticisms, and observations on how to flesh out the details of how best to improve HSAs through this hearing.

Now I will yield to Mr. Thompson for the purpose of an opening statement.

Mr. Thompson. Thank you, Mr. Chairman. Thank you for holding the hearing.

And thanks to the witnesses for being here today.

As it stands today, high-deductible health plans and the health savings accounts that accompany them plug a gap in the market. They offer employers a lower cost alternative amid ever-climbing large and small group coverage rates and give patients a hand in making out-of-pocket payments. These plans are a reflection of a healthcare market where cost growth continues to place quality care out of reach for far too many people.

Health spending grows at more than two times the rate of inflation. In the employer market, this is a direct result of the cost of care, including factors such as prescription drugs or hospital inpatient stays. No one player in the healthcare industry is without some responsibility for these increasing costs.

As policymakers, our reaction must not be to incentivize the shift of those costs to consumers. It is not a cost containment solution; it is a cop-out. It doesn't address the root of the problem, it is not sustainable, and it doesn't help the people that we represent, because forcing patients to feel the pain of their care cost doesn't necessarily lead patients to choose treatments that drive the best possible outcomes.

At the end of the day, patients are not expert consumers of healthcare, and simply exposing them to high prices doesn't change their understanding of the value of a treatment, what gets them the most bang for their buck. That is in large part because they may not have a choice given the consolidation or provider affiliations, or they simply don't have the time, expertise, nor information to become truly well informed.

In California, for example, hospitals report charges for their 25 most common outpatient procedures, but that information isn't standardized or audited for accuracy. California Healthcare Compare, the State's online tool for consumers to compare price and quality, offers only that information which insurers and providers have elected to share.

Options that look appropriate based on the site's information may not even be in the patient's high-deductible health plan's network. And for the quarter of consumers enrolled in high-deductible health plans, all the information in the world isn't going to help them meet their deductible when they have no HSA and their out-of-pocket costs are simply unaffordable.

From our witnesses today we can learn more about the technical aspects of these plans, how we remedy unintended consequences of existing policies, and the impact of changes, like those sought by members of our committee on a bipartisan basis. But we should be under no false impression that such change will provide our constituents with meaningful relief from the type of healthcare bills that leave them deciding between rent and critical care.

This committee has more work to do to address growing healthcare costs, and I look forward to working with my colleagues to develop and improve policies set forth under the ACA to bend the cost curve over the long term.

Mr. Chairman, is now the appropriate time for me to introduce the Democratic witness?

Chairman Roskam. Not quite yet, but it is coming soon.

Mr. Thompson. But you will let me know?

Chairman Roskam. Yes, sir.

Mr. Thompson. All right. Thank you. I yield back.

Chairman Roskam. Thank you, Mr. Thompson.

Without objection, any member's opening statements will be made part of the record.

We will hear from our witnesses. Let me briefly introduce three of them and then I will yield to Mr. Thompson.

First, we will hear from Roy Ramthun, who is the president and founder of Ask Mr. HSA Service, who will give us an account and basically an overview of the creation of HSAs and explain the benefits of consumer-directed healthcare and why access to these accounts should be expanded.

Next, we will hear from Matt Eyles, the president and CEO of AHIP, America's Health Insurance Plans, who will update us on the enrollment trends and demographics of account holders. His testimony is going to highlight some of the experience of HSAs in the individual market, including the exchanges and how HSAs can offer lower costs for middle-income Americans.

Then we will hear from Jody Dietel, who is the chief compliance officer at WageWorks, who is going to present data that will inform us about who will be benefiting from HSAs today. In addition, she will give us insight on the barriers that employers are facing when they try to offer these plans.

And now I would yield to Mr. Thompson for the introduction of our final witness.

Mr. Thompson. Thank you, Mr. Chairman.

And thank you, Dr. Sherry Glied, for being with us today.

Dr. Glied currently serves as the dean of New York University's Robert F. Wagner Graduate School of Public Service. Prior to her work in academia, Dr. Glied served as the Assistant Secretary for Planning and Evaluation at HHS, and she was a member of the President's Council of Economic Advisers.

As an expert on the intersection of healthcare and economics, Dr. Glied can provide our committee with valuable insight on how we can most effectively address cost and affordability in the context of consumer-directed accounts.

Dr. Glied, thank you for being with us.

Chairman Roskam. Thank you all for being with us today. As I explained in a little pregame a moment ago, each of you have 5 minutes. Your written testimony is a part of the record, and this committee is familiar with it.

Then we will invite members to inquire. n old trick is for members to talk for about 4-1/2 minutes and then use 15 seconds to pose a question and then give you 5 seconds to answer. So we will try and resist that temptation today.

And, Mr. Ramthun, we will start with you. You are recognized.

STATEMENT OF ROY RAMTHUN, PRESIDENT AND FOUNDER, HSA CONSULTING SERVICES, LLC

Mr. Ramthun. Thank you.

Chairman Roskam, Ranking Member Levin, and members of the subcommittee, I thank you for this opportunity to testify before you today. My name is Roy Ramthun, and I led the implementation of the HSA program after its enactment in 2003 while serving at the U.S. Treasury Department.

A few years later, I started my own consulting practice to devote my full time and attention to this program and related issues.

The HSA market is currently dominated by employer-sponsored coverage, with over 80 percent of the enrollment coming from large employers. Employee enrollment in high-deductible health plans has doubled over the past 6 years, with approximately 30 percent of employees now being enrolled in these plans, many of whom have HSAs.

I expect these trends to continue as long as premiums increase faster than inflation and the ACA's Cadillac plan tax looms in the future.

In contrast, the individual market was originally the largest source of HSAs, but over time has fallen to under 10 percent of all participants.

HSA plans have been available on the State health insurance exchanges since 2014, primarily as Bronze and Silver Plans. But as with the rest of the individual market, carrier exits and reduced product offerings have limited HSA plan choices more recently.

Regardless of market segment, it seems as if every plan is a high-deductible plan today, but not all plans with high deductibles make individuals eligible for HSAs. Recent data from the National Center for Health Statistics indicates that approximately 43 percent of working age adults are enrolled in high-deductible health plans, but only about 18 percent are enrolled in an HSA-qualified plan, leaving the other 25 percent without access to an HSA.

As a result, millions of Americans face similar exposure to out-of-pocket costs but cannot use an HSA to protect them.

HSAs could be a part of the solution to this problem. HSAs require no guesswork and no reason to fear losing the money that is not spent each year. In fact, most people could save money simply by adding up all their qualified health expenses at the end of the year and reimbursing them through their HSA.

There are numerous legislative proposals to modify HSAs pending before the Ways and Means Committee, including bills introduced by members of this subcommittee. In particular, I would like to acknowledge the leadership of Representative Erik Paulsen, who has sponsored the Health Savings Act for the past several Congresses.

The HSA industry still considers this bill the gold standard for HSA legislation. I have summarized and categorized the legislation as part of my written testimony for your review.

I believe the simplest way to allow more Americans to access HSAs is to move to a more flexible health plan design based on actuarial value. Actuarial value tells us how generous a plan's benefit design is based on its deductibles, copays, coinsurance, and annual out-of-pocket limits.

For example, an actuarial value of 90 percent indicates that a plan is designed to cover 90 percent of the benefit costs on average, leaving 10 percent to be paid out-of-pocket by the enrollees. Since deductibles and out-of-pocket limits have the greatest impact on actuarial value, plans with lower deductibles and lower out-of-pocket limits typically have higher actuarial values.

Actuarial value could become an alternative way of determining HSA eligibility. I recommend that health plans with actuarial values below 80 percent also make consumers eligible for HSAs.

I believe 80 percent is a reasonable standard because HSA-qualified plans can currently be offered in the gold metal tier on the State insurance exchanges, and I also believe employer-sponsored coverage is close to 80 percent currently.

I hope you will consider this proposal as you contemplate making changes to HSAs.

In conclusion, I support expanding HSAs to more Americans to help them with their growing out-of-pocket costs. I also support expanding contribution limits for HSAs so that everyone has the opportunity to cover their full risk for out-of-pocket expenses through their HSA. This would especially help Americans with chronic conditions and high medical bills.

Mr. Chairman and members of the subcommittee, I appreciate the opportunity to provide this testimony today. I look forward to discussing these issues in greater detail with you, and I would be pleased to answer any questions you have. Thank you.

Written Statement of Roy J. Ramthun, President, HSA Consulting Services, LLC, before the Subcommittee on Health Committee on Ways and Means, U.S. House of Representatives, Wednesday, June 6, 2018

Chairman Roskam, Ranking Member Levin and members of the Subcommittee, I would like to thank you for this opportunity to testify before the Subcommittee on Health about how consumer-directed health plans and Health Savings Accounts (HSAs) can help lower costs and expand access to health care. My name is Roy Ramthun, and I am a private consultant residing in the Washington, DC area. My consulting practice focuses primarily on helping financial institutions, HSA administrators, employers, health plans, brokers, and consumers to better understand and take advantage of the benefits offered by consumer-driven health care programs such as HSAs and their associated health insurance plans.

I have had the distinct honor to serve our country in positions at the U.S. Senate Committee on Finance, the White House, the Treasury Department, and the Department of Health and Human Services (HHS). While at the Treasury Department, I led the implementation of the HSA program after its enactment in 2003. I started my own consulting practice after leaving the White House in 2006 to devote my full time and attention to this program and related issues.

Brief History of HSAs

HSAs were officially created in the Medicare Modernization Act of 2003 (P.L.: 108-173), although they can trace their roots to a demonstration program created in the Health Insurance Portability and Accountability Act (HIPAA) of 1996 (P.L. 104–191) known as Archer Medical Savings Accounts (MSAs). The basic structure has remained largely unchanged since 2003, with somewhat modest changes having been made in the Health Opportunity Patient Empowerment (HOPE) Act of 2006 (title III of P.L. 109-432) and the Affordable Care Act of 2010 (P.L. 111–148). Starting in 2014, HSA-qualified health insurance plans have been offered on the state health insurance exchanges as well.

Evolution of HSAs Since 2003

The history of the HSA program is a tale of two markets. In the early days, most of the growth in HSAs came from individuals and small employers. Over time, larger employers have driven most of the growth, according to data from America's Health Insurance Plans (see Figure 1 below). According to the National Business Group on Health, nine in ten employers (90%) will offer at least one consumer-driven health plan in 2018. In addition, nearly forty percent (40%) of employers will offer a consumer-driven health plan as the only plan option in 2018, compared with thirty-five percent (35%) in 2017.

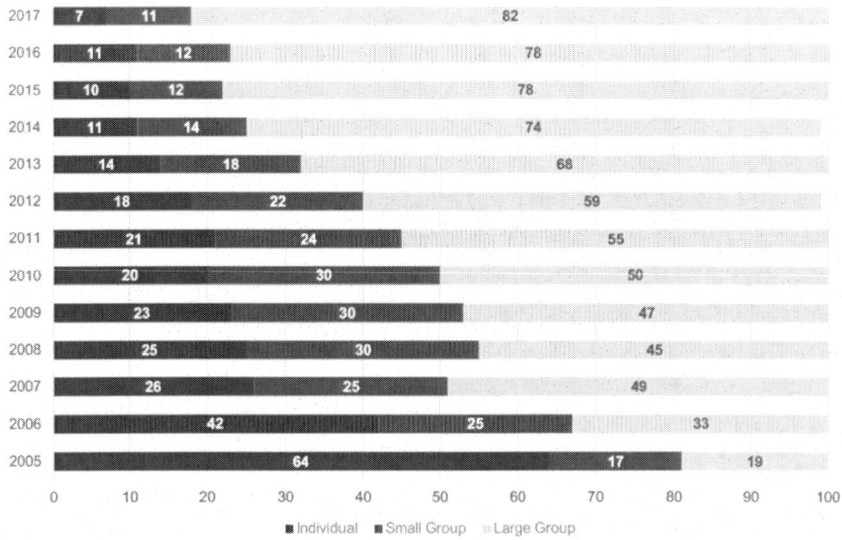

Figure 1. Percentage of Individuals in the Commercial Health Insurance Market Covered by an HSA-Qualified High-Deductible Health Plan, by Market Type, 2005-2017.

The most common consumer-driven plan design is a high-deductible health plan paired with an HSA, offered by eighty percent (80%) of employers with any type of consumer-driven health plan. Today, consumer-driven health plans are the fastest growing product in the market for employer- based group health plans. Estimates vary, but approximately thirty percent (30%) of employees are now enrolled in consumer-driven health plans. This percentage has doubled over the past 6 years. What is fueling the growth in consumer-driven health plans? One of the reasons is the dramatic increase in health insurance premiums (see Figure 2 below).

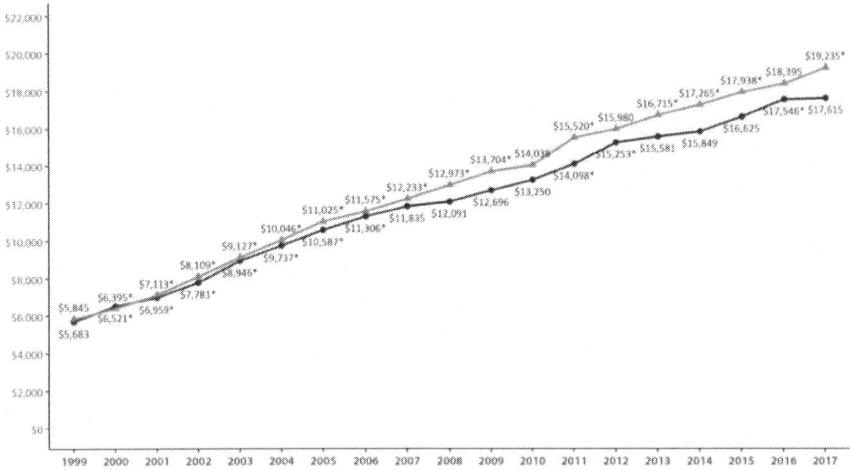

* Estimate is statistically different from estimate for the previous year shown (p<.05).
Source: Kaiser/HRET Survey of Employer Sponsored Health Benefits, 1999-2017.

Figure 2. Average Annual Premiums for Covered Workers with Family Coverage, by Firm Size, 1999-2017.

Other surveys suggest that costs may be even higher. For example, Milliman Inc. recently reported that health care costs for the typical family of four are projected to reach $28,166 through an employer-sponsored preferred provider organization (PPO) plan this year. The 4.5 percent increase in projected costs for 2018 is the second lowest in the 18-year history of Milliman's Medical Index, just slightly above last year's record low rate of 4.3 percent.

As premiums have risen, employers and insurance carriers have increased deductibles almost annually in an effort to moderate year-over-year premium increases. Fifteen years ago, it was hard to find high deductible plans in the large employer group market. Today, it seems as if every plan is a high deductible plan as deductibles for preferred provider organizations (PPOs) and even health maintenance organizations (HMOs) have risen to levels similar to that for HSAs. Annual deductibles for workers with employer-sponsored HSA plans averaged $2,433 for self-only coverage, and $4,647 for family coverage in 2017.[1]

Issues, Challenges and Opportunities for HSAs

HSA eligibility requires enrollment in a high deductible health insurance plan. But not all plans with high deductibles make individuals eligible for HSAs. This is due to the strict requirements for "HSA-qualified" high deductible plans. At the beginning of the program (2004), this meant a deductible of $1,000 for self-only coverage and $2,000 for family coverage. The minimum deductibles are adjusted annually for inflation[2] and have increased modestly since 2004. For 2018, the minimum deductibles have risen to $1,350 for self-only coverage and $2,700 for family coverage. If a health insurance plan does not meet the minimum deductible for 2018, it cannot be an HSA-qualified plan. While other plans may have deductibles above these amounts, there are other reasons why they are not HSA-qualified.

One of the main features that separates HSA-qualified plans from other health insurance plans with high deductibles is that the HSA-qualified plan deductible must apply to all covered benefits, including prescription drugs, received from in-network providers. Plans that do not apply a deductible or apply a separate lower deductible to prescription drugs cannot be an HSA-

---

[1] Kaiser Family Foundation, "2017 Employer Health Benefits Survey," September 19, 2017, Figure 8.7, https://www.kff.org/report-section/ehbs-2017-section-8-high-deductible-health-plans-with-savings-option/.

[2] Initially, the inflation adjustment factor was the consumer price index (CPI) but this has now been changed to chained-CPI as a result of the tax reform law enacted in December 2017.

qualified plan. The only benefits that may be covered before the deductible is met are preventive care services. In 2010, the Affordable Care Act borrowed this concept from HSAs and made coverage of preventive care services a requirement for all health plans regardless of deductible, including self-insured employer-sponsored plans.

Another key requirement for HSA-qualified plans is an annual limit on out-of-pocket expenses. At the beginning of the program (2004), this meant annual limits of no more than $5,000 for self- only coverage and $10,000 for family coverage. The annual out-of-pocket limits are also adjusted annually for inflation[3] and have increased modestly since 2004. For 2018, these amounts have risen to $6,650 for self-only coverage and $13,300 for family coverage. If a health insurance plan does not limit annual out-of-pocket expenses to these or lower amounts for 2018, it cannot be an HSA-qualified plan.

Annual out-of-pocket limits are another feature borrowed from HSAs by the Affordable Care Act (ACA) which made them a requirement for all health plans, including self-insured employer- sponsored plans. In 2014, the ACA out-of-pocket limits started out at the same amounts as the HSA out-of-pocket limits. But the annual inflation adjustment factor used to adjust the ACA limits is the medical component of the consumer price index (M-CPI) whereas the HSA- qualified plans limits have since been adjusted by CPI (now chained-CPI). Thus, the ACA out- of-pocket limits have risen much faster than the HSA limits. For example, for 2018 the ACA out-of-pocket limits are $7,350 for self-only coverage and $14,700 for family coverage, $700 and $1,400 higher than the HSA limits, respectively. This means that HSA-qualified plans provide better protection against high medical expenses than the ACA requires. Further, all plans with annual out-of-pocket limits above the HSA-qualified limits deny their enrollees access to an HSA which could greatly help them pay for their out-of-pocket costs.

There isn't much information regarding how high employers offering self-insured health plans are setting their annual out-of-pocket limits. In the

---

[3] Ibid.

individual market, the picture is clearer. According to an analysis by Ed Haislmaier of the Heritage Foundation, more than half of all plan designs (54.7 percent) in the 39 states using the federally run exchange through Healthcare.gov set out-of-pocket limits at the maximum allowed by the ACA.[4] Cost-sharing limits are set at the maximum level allowed for:

- all Catastrophic-level plans
- 51 percent of Bronze-level plan designs
- 58 percent of Silver-level plan designs
- 41 percent of Gold-level plan designs.

Because the ACA's maximum out-of-pocket limits are higher than those for HSA-qualified plans, over half (57 percent) of all plan designs now offered through the federal exchange have out-of-pocket maximums that are too high for the plan to qualify for an HSA. As shown in Chart 1 below, only 30 percent of plans sold on the federal exchange meet the criteria of having both a deductible high enough and an out-of-pocket limit low enough to qualify for an HSA. Of the plans that are not HSA-qualified, 19 percent fail to qualify because their deductibles are too low, while 81 percent do not qualify because their out-of-pocket limits are too high.[5]

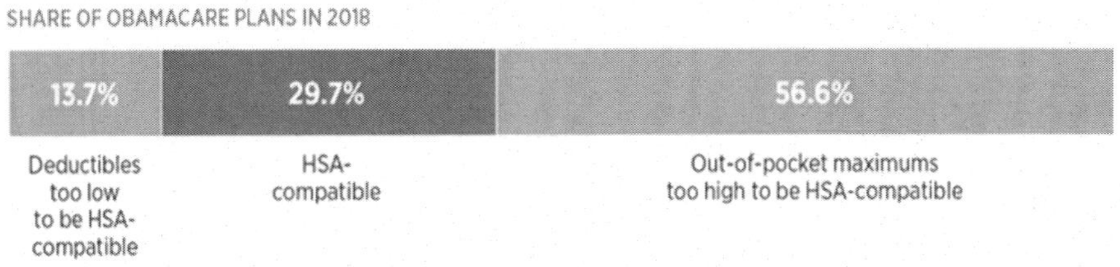

Source: Author;s calculations based on data from HHS Individual Market Landscape from Healthcare.gov. IB4862. Heritage.org.

Chart 1. Few Obamacare Plans Are HAS-Compatible.

---

[4] "Obamacare's Cost Sharing is Too High, Even for HSAs," https://www.heritage.org/health-care- r eform/report/obamacares-cost-sharing-too-high-even-hsas.

[5] Ibid.

Under most of ACA's HSA-qualified plan designs, annual deductibles exceed the maximum amount that an individual could contribute to their HSA. Of the HSA-qualified plan designs offered in the 39 Healthcare.gov states, 52 percent have deductibles for self-only coverage that are higher than the maximum HSA contribution amount of $3,450, and 61 percent have deductibles for family coverage that are higher than the maximum HSA contribution amount of $6,900. One-quarter of the HSA-qualified plan designs have deductibles set at, or near, the maximum out-of-pocket limit.

In the first few years of the state insurance exchanges, HSA-qualified plans were generally available, primarily in the Silver and Bronze metal tiers. But carrier exits and reductions in plan offerings have also impacted HSAs. In 2018, six of the 39 states using the federal exchange have counties in which no HSA-qualified plans are available, including Pennsylvania and Tennessee (see Table 1).[6]

Table 1. States with counties that do not have any HAS-Compatible plans on the exchange

		Counties without HSA-Compatible Plans	
State	Total Counties	Number	Percent
Missouri	115	7	6%
Ohio	88	6	7%
Oklahoma	77	20	26%
Pennsylvania	67	20	30%
Tennessee	95	5	5%
Virginia	134	13	10%

Source: Author's calculations based on data from HHS Individual Market Landscape from Healthcare.gov.

[6] Edmund F. Haislmaier, "2018 Obamacare Health Insurance Exchanges: Competition and Choice Continue to Shrink," Heritage Foundation Issue Brief No. 4813, January 25, 2018, https://www.heritage.org/sites/default/files/2018-01/IB4813_1.pdf.

Looking more broadly at American's health insurance coverage throughout the year, recent data from the National Center for Health Statistics indicates that enrollment in consumer-driven health plans has grown by about seventy percent (70%) over the past seven years. Enrollment in HSA-qualified plans has doubled during this same time. Despite this growth, many more Americans are enrolled in other plans with high deductibles that do not make them eligible for an HSA. I will address this disparity later in my testimony.

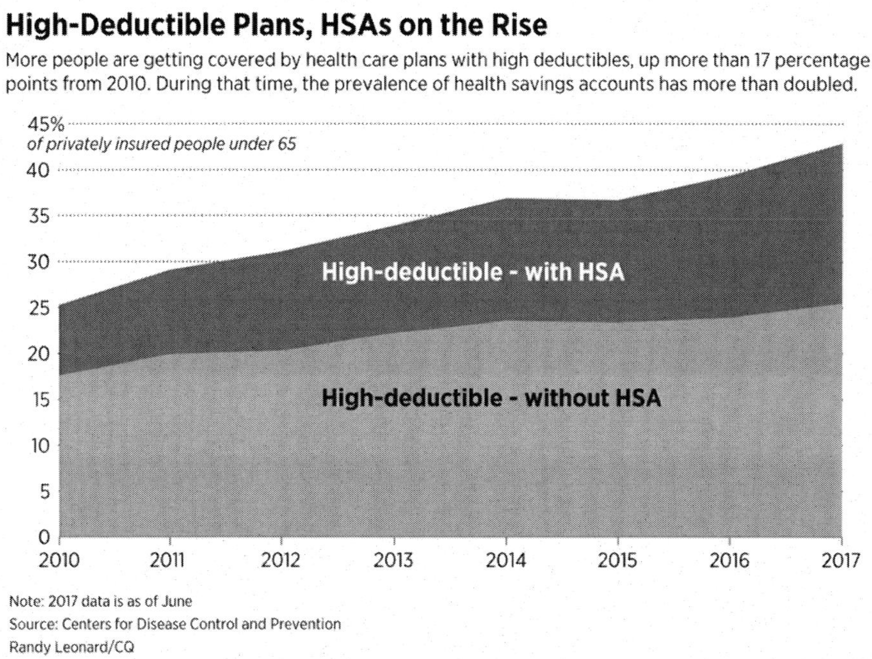

Figure 3.

The Benefits of Consumer-Driven Health Care

There are several benefits of consumer-driven health care, including premium savings for employers and workers, lower year-over-year trend, tax-free contributions by employers to workers' HSAs, and more engaged consumers. I will address each of these benefits below.

Premium Savings for Employers

One of the biggest reasons employers are switching to HSAs is because the premiums are about $2,400 less than traditional plans for family coverage, as can be seen from the table below (Figure 4) from the September 2017 report by the Kaiser Family Foundation/Health Research in Education Trust (KFF/HRET).[7] Employers could just pocket their savings, but this chapter indicates that many of them are sharing their premium savings with their workers in the form of contributions to workers' HSAs. On average this amounts to $1,100 per worker for those with family coverage.

	Single Coverage			Family Coverage		
	HDHP/HRA	HSA-Qualified HDHP	Non-HDHP/SO Plans	HDHP/HRA	HSA-Qualified HDHP	Non-HDHP/SO Plans
Annual Premium	$6,438*	$5,773*	$6,949	$18,948	$16,821*	$19,225
Worker Contribution to Premium	$1,216	$918*	$1,288	$5,130*	$4,289*	$6,149
Firm Contribution to Premium	$5,222	$4,855*	$5,661	$13,817	$12,532	$13,076
Annual Firm Contribution to the HRA or HSA	$1,351	$608	Not Applicable	$2,444	$1,086	Not Applicable
Total Annual Firm Contribution (Firm Share of Premium Plus Firm Contribution to HRA or HSA)	$6,573*	$5,473	$5,661	$16,261*	$13,608	$13,076
Total Annual Cost (Total Premium Plus Firm Contribution to HRA or HSA)	**$7,789***	**$6,390***	**$6,949**	**$21,391***	**$17,895***	**$19,225**

NOTE: When those firms that do not contribute to the HSA (47% for single coverage and 46% for family coverage) are excluded from the calculation, the average firm contribution to the HSA for covered workers is $795 for single coverage and $1,417 for family coverage. Three percent of covered workers are enrolled in a plan where the firm matches employee HSA contributions. For HDHP/HRAs, we refer to the amount that the employer commits to make available to an HRA as a contribution for ease of discussion. HRAs are notional accounts, and employers are not required to actually transfer funds until an employee incurs expenses. Thus, employers may not expend the entire amount that they commit to make available to their employees through an HRA. Covered workers enrolled in a plan where the firm matches any employee contribution to an HSA account are not included in the average contribution (3% for single coverage and 3% for family coverage). Values shown in the table may not equal the sum of their component parts. The averages presented in the table are aggregated at the firm level and then averaged, which is methodologically more appropriate than adding the averages.

* Estimate is statistically different from estimate for Non-HDHP/SO Plans ($p < .05$).

SOURCE: Kaiser/HRET Survey of Employer-Sponsored Health Benefits, 2017

Figure 4. Average Annual Premiums and Contributions to Savings Accounts for Covered Workers in HDHP/HRAs or HSA-Qualified HDHPs, Compared to Non-HDHP/SO Plans, 2017.

According to Willis Towers Watson's 22nd annual Best Practices in Health Care Employer Survey,[8] seventy-seven percent (77%) of best performing companies have moved their employees into consumer-driven health plans. Combined with other strategies, this has led to significant savings on their health benefit costs. Best-performing companies achieved

[7] https://www.kff.org/health-costs/report/2017-employer-health-benefits-survey/.

[8] https://www.willistowerswatson.com/en/press/2018/03/best-performing-companies-achieve-significant-health- c are-cost-savings.

a $2,251 per employee per year health care cost advantage over the national average in 2017 ($9,950 compared with $12,201). Other studies have shown similar results. This is hard evidence of "bending the cost curve" that is so elusive for the rest of our nation's health care system.

Why isn't every company offering consumer-driven health plans? They may have to if the ACA's "Cadillac plan" tax ever goes into effect. Companies may have few other options as effective as consumer-driven health plans to keep their costs below the thresholds where the excise tax will affect them.

Premium Savings for Employees

Not only are employers saving money on premiums, workers are too – approximately $1,850 for family coverage (see Figure 8.8 above), according to the 2017 report from KFF/HRET.

Employer Contributions to Employees' HSAs

Employers could just pocket their premium savings, but the 2017 KFF/HRET report indicates that many of them are sharing their premium savings with their workers in the form of contributions to workers' HSAs. On average this amounts to $1,100 per worker for those with family coverage. Combined with workers' own premium savings of $1,850, almost $3,000 can be deposited in their HSAs without taking money away from their retirement plan, take-home pay or other savings.

Lower Overall Spending on Health Care

The potential for bending the cost curve for national health care spending was confirmed several years ago when researchers at the RAND Corporation published in the journal *Health Affairs* the results of their analysis of the potential impact of consumer-driven health plans on the American health care system.[9] The RAND analysis suggested that if consumer-driven health plans grow to represent half of all employer-sponsored insurance in the United States, health care spending could drop

[9] https://www.rand.org/pubs/research_briefs/RB9690z3/index1.html.

by \$57 billion annually—about 4 percent of all health care spending among non- elderly Americans. The study acknowledges that HSAs are far more cost-effective and estimates that if all of the same people were covered by HSA-qualified plans the annual savings would be as high as \$73.6 billion. This may be a conservative estimate.

More Engaged Consumers

But consumer-driven health plans are not just about saving money. It's also about *how* the money is saved—by changing how employees think about their health and taking action to improve it. I would like to take a few moments to clear up some common misperceptions about consumer-driven health plans.

First, research is increasingly suggesting that lifestyle behaviors account for approximately three- quarters of health care spending in the U.S. This is likely to only get worse as diet, obesity, lack of exercise, and smoking take its toll on our bodies and our health care system. Fortunately, consumer-driven health plans cover preventive care services without applying a deductible or other out-of-pocket expense. In fact, "free" preventive care was included in the original design of HSAs, long before the ACA made it a requirement of all health plans. Data from Aetna, Cigna, the Employee Benefit Research Institute (EBRI), and others suggests that utilization of preventive care services is higher when individuals are enrolled in consumer-driven health plans. Additional data suggests higher compliance with disease management and treatment regimens for individuals with chronic conditions. While there is always a risk that people will seek less care when spending their own money (several studies have raised this concern), I am not aware of any evidence to suggest that the health status of individuals enrolled in consumer-driven health plans has declined, and in most cases, it appears to be improving. Obviously, this is an issue to monitor for the future.

Second, individuals enrolled in consumer-driven health plans are more engaged in their health care. Several surveys by EBRI suggest that enrollees in consumer-driven health plans are more likely to: (1) check whether their plan would cover their care; (2) talk to their doctor about treatment options and costs; (3) talk to their doctor about prescription drug options and costs; (4) ask for a generic drug; (5) check the price of service before seeking care; (6) use an online cost-tracking tool; and (7) develop a budget to manage health care expenses. Similar findings have been reported by insurance carriers.

Third, HSA-qualified consumer-driven health plans provide true catastrophic protection by virtue of their annual limits on out-of-pocket expenses and have been doing so since 2004. These limits apply both to medical and pharmacy expenses and therefore provide an extremely important benefit to people with chronic conditions and/or high annual health care expenses.

Fourth, covered benefits and services are generally identical to traditional plans, not "skimpier" as some critics believe. The ACA does not allow it except for other types of insurance plans which are not generally HSA-qualified. What is different is the amount of covered benefits paid by the consumer-driven health plan. So, while the exact same benefits may be covered by each plan, the consumer-driven health plan may only cover 60 or 70 percent of the cost of covered benefits, whereas a traditional HMO or PPO plan may cover 80 or 90 percent of the cost of covered benefits, on average. However, the difference in out-of-pocket costs for covered benefits is typically offset almost dollar-for-dollar by a difference in premiums. For example, a plan with a higher deductible (by $2,000) will typically have a premium that is $2,000 lower. Many people understand this concept when applied to their auto and homeowner's insurance policies, but the concept is still relatively new to many people for their health insurance.

Fifth, even though individuals enrolled in consumer-driven health plans typically have higher out-of-pocket expenses, they still receive the benefit of the discounted prices for medical services negotiated by their insurance plan. For example, a patient may have an office visit with his or her personal physician. While the physician may charge $150 for each office visit, he/she usually accepts a discounted fee of $70 to $100 depending on the insurance plan. In these cases, the patient would pay only

$70 to $100 until their deductible is met, not the full $150 charged by the physician.

Sixth, there is a growing industry of companies providing transparency services to help people manage their medical care and health care finances. Companies like Compass, Medibid, BidRx, ZendyHealth, Healthcare Blue Book, and others are responding to the needs of patients by providing better information about the price and quality of health care services. Another industry is responding to the demand for "wellness" services to help people maintain and improve their health to avoid disease and chronic conditions. These companies would likely not exist without the growing consumer demand for better value for their health care dollar.

Finally, even though individuals enrolled in consumer-driven health plans are typically subject to higher up-front deductibles, most employers are providing a contribution of funds to the associated HSA which helps lessen the sting of the deductible. In addition, workers' premium savings can also be re-directed towards funding their HSAs. With HSAs, unspent funds automatically accumulate each year and are therefore available to meet future health expenses.

Why HSAs Should Be Expanded

Eligibility for HSAs should be expanded so that millions more Americans can take advantage of their protection against high out-of-pocket costs. As deductibles have risen dramatically for all plans since the enactment of the Affordable Care Act, there is a greater need for helping Americans save for their out-of-pocket costs. HSAs could be part of the solution to this problem. HSAs are not limited to workers with the right employment – anyone that is eligible can establish and contribute to an HSA. In addition, there is no guesswork involved and no reason to fear losing the money that is not spent each year. In fact, most people could save money simply by adding up all their qualified health expenses at the end of the year and reimbursing them through their HSA.

Proposals to Expand/Modify HSAs

Currently, there are numerous legislative proposals to modify HSAs, including some bipartisan legislation. The industry-supported "gold standard" is the Health Savings Act (H.R. 1175) sponsored by Health Subcommittee member Rep. Erik Paulsen (R-MN).

In general, HSA-related bills seek to do one or more of the following:

1. Make more Americans eligible for HSAs;
2. Allow Americans to contribute more money to their HSAs each year;
3. Allow HSAs to be more flexible so funds can be used for additional health-related expenses;
4. Allow HSA assets to be transferred or rolled over tax-free to a child, parent, or grandparent of an account owner (currently limited to spouses); or
5. Protect HSA assets from creditors in personal bankruptcy situations.

I have attached a summary of the bills introduced in the 115th Congress that include provisions addressing each of these areas (see Attachment 1).

Moving to a More Flexible Plan Design for HSAs

After reviewing the existing legislative proposals, I believe the simplest way to allow more Americans to access HSAs is to move to a more flexible health plan design for HSA-eligibility instead of the rigid "high deductible health plan" with all its bells and whistles. Americans don't want to hear why they can't have an HSA. They want to know how they can take advantage of an HSA, too.

I recently wrote a white paper[10] about one approach towards moving to a more flexible plan design based on actuarial value instead of specific deductibles and other requirements. Actuarial value is a numerical value that reflects the generosity of the plan's coverage. For example, a plan with an actuarial value of eighty percent (80%) is designed to cover eighty percent (80%) of the cost of the benefits covered by the plan, on average, leaving 20 percent to be paid out-of- pocket by the individual(s) enrolled in the plan.

Actuarial value reflects the plan design features including deductibles, copays, coinsurance, and annual limits on out-of-pocket expenses. In general, the greater the amount of covered benefits the plan pays (i.e., the less the consumer pays out-of-pocket), the higher the actuarial value. Since deductibles and out-of-pocket limits have the greatest impact on actuarial value, this means that plans with lower deductibles and lower out-of-pocket limits typically have higher actuarial values because the plan pays a larger share of the total benefit costs. Conversely, plans with higher deductibles and higher out-of-pocket limits typically have lower actuarial values because the plan pays a smaller share of the total benefit costs.

Actuarial value is a common calculation in insurance plan design but is not typically known by or disclosed to consumers except for the "metal tier plans" (e.g., Bronze, Silver, etc.) available in the state health insurance exchanges under the ACA. Actuarial value can help consumers compare the cost of premiums relative to their exposure for out-of-pocket costs. Under the ACA, insurance carriers use a standardized methodology (the "AV Calculator") for determining the actuarial value of each plan offered on the state insurance exchanges in a standardized way. This methodology or a similar standard could be used for this purpose.

In my white paper, I propose that future HSA eligibility could be based on a plan's actuarial value instead of specific deductibles and other plan features. I recommend that enrollment in a health plan with an actuarial value below eighty percent (80%) would make consumers eligible for an HSA. I recommend this threshold for actuarial value because HSA-

---

[10] https://www.aba.com/Advocacy/Issues/Documents/Moving-More-Flexible-Standard-HSAs.pdf.

qualified plans can currently be offered in the Gold metal tier on the state insurance exchanges.

Once an AV standard is set for future HSA-qualified plans, insurance carriers should have the flexibility to design plans with vary levels of cost-sharing. All plans with actuarial values below the eighty percent (80%) threshold would make consumers eligible for HSAs. Plans with actuarial values above that standard would not. I hope you will consider this proposal as you contemplate making changes to HSAs.

Conclusion

I support expanding HSAs to more Americans to help them with their growing out-of-pocket costs. I also support expanding contribution limits for HSAs so that everyone has the opportunity to cover their risk of out-of-pocket expenses through their HSA. One never knows when a "really bad year" might be lurking around the corner. If we are lucky enough to keep our job and our health, then the money we save will help us pay for our health care in retirement. With Medicare's finances less than certain and the potential cost of long term care, expanding HSAs is one way of helping us all.

On another Medicare-related note, when I turn 65 I will not have the option to stay off Medicare even if I continue to work as a self-employed individual. I think this should be changed. I would like to continue my HSA eligibility and save taxpayers money by not having Medicare cover my medical bills until I fully retire. Expanding HSAs to working seniors would eliminate the discrimination for millions of pre-retirees that can and choose to work beyond age 65. Many of us want to and have the incentive to do so because we will not be able to qualify for full Social Security benefits until age 67.

Mr. Chairman and members of the Subcommittee, I appreciate the opportunity to provide this testimony today. I look forward to the opportunity to discuss these issues in greater detail with you. I would be pleased to answer any questions you have.

Thank you.

ATTACHMENT 1. HSA-RELATED LEGISLATION INTRODUCED IN THE 115TH CONGRESS, AS OF JUNE 1, 2018

- Bills that Would Make More Americans Eligible for HSAs
  - Deem all Bronze, Silver, and Catastrophic plans sold on the state insurance exchanges as HSA-qualified plans – H.R. 35 (Burgess)
  - Eliminate the requirement that an HSA-eligible individual be enrolled in an HSA- qualified plan – H.R. 247 (Brat), H.R. 408 (King), H.R. 1072 (Sanford)
  - Clarify that direct primary care services are not "insurance" that would disqualify an individual from HSA eligibility – H.R. 365 (Paulsen), H.R. 1175 (Paulsen), H.R. 1280 (Fortenberry)
  - Allow Medicare beneficiaries to contribute to an HSA – H.R. 408 (King).
  - Allow HSA-eligible seniors enrolled in Medicare Part A only to contribute to HSAs – H.R. 1175 (Paulsen)
  - Allow Native Americans that are otherwise HSA-eligible to contribute to their HSAs regardless of utilization of IHS or tribal medical services – H.R. 1175 (Paulsen), H.R. 1476 (Moolenaar)
  - Allow members of health care sharing ministries to contribute to HSAs – H.R. 1175 (Paulsen), H.R. 2310 (Kelly)

- o Allow HSA-eligible individuals to receive specified health care services at their employer's on-site medical clinic without cancelling their HSA-eligibility – H.R. 1175 (Paulsen)
- o Allow HSA-eligible health plans to use embedded deductibles for family coverage that are as low as the minimum deductible for self-only coverage (i.e., $1,300/person vs. $2,600/person for 2017) – H.R. 1175 (Paulsen)
- o Expand the definition of "preventive care" services to include certain prescription and over-the-counter drugs for chronic conditions – H.R. 1175 (Paulsen)
- o Modify the safe harbor definition of "preventive care" to include care related to the treatment of any medically complex chronic condition – H.R. 4978 (Black/Blumenauer), H.R. 5138 (Kelly)
- o Modify the definition of "permitted insurance" that HSA-eligible individuals may have coverage under without impacting their HSA eligibility to include insurance policies known as "excepted benefits" – H.R. 5138 (Kelly)
- o Allow HSA-eligible workers to access certain medical services provided at on-site employer clinics or retail clinics without impacting their HSA eligibility – H.R. 5138 (Kelly)
- o Allow otherwise HSA-eligible individuals to contribute to their HSA even when their spouse participates in a general health FSA – H.R. 5138 (Kelly)
- o Allow individuals participating in a health FSA or HRA to become HSA-eligible if unused funds in the FSA or HRA are converted to a post-deductible FSA or HRA, a limited purpose FSA or HRA, a retirement HRA, a suspended HRA, or the remaining FSA or HRA funds are used solely for preventive care – H.R. 5138 (Kelly)
- o Allow individuals to disclaim any coverage that would disqualify them from HSA eligibility – H.R. 5138 (Kelly)

  - o Modify the definition of an HSA-qualified plan to permit coverage of two primary care office visits before the deductible is satisfied (H.R. 5858)
- Bills that Would Allow Americans to Contribute More Money to Their HSAs
  - o Set the maximum contribution to an HSA at the annual limit for out-of-pocket expenses under an HSA-qualified plan (i.e., $6,650 for singles, $13,300 for families for 2018) – H.R. 35 (Burgess), H.R. 1175 (Paulsen), H.R. 1280 (Fortenberry), H.R. 1628 (Black), H.R. 4200 (Brady)
  - o Increase the HSA annual contribution limits to $10,000 singles and $20,000 families – H.R. 408 (King).
  - o Remove the maximum annual contribution limit to HSAs (i.e., unlimited contributions to HSAs permitted) – H.R. 1072 (Sanford)
  - o Allow an additional tax deduction for amounts contributed to the HSA of a taxpayer's child or grandchild – H.R. 35 (Burgess)
  - o Allow taxpayers to establish HSAs for their minor children and contribute up to $3,000 to each child's HSA (contributions are tax deductible) – H.R. 277 (Roe)
  - o Eliminate the need to pro-rate contributions for partial year eligibility – H.R. 408 (King)
  - o Change the inflation adjustment for contribution limits to medical CPI – H.R. 408 (King).
  - o Add an annual inflation adjustment to the catch-up contribution limit – H.R. 408 (King).
  - o Allow both spouses to make catch-up contributions to the same HSA account – H.R. 1175 (Paulsen), H.R. 1628 (Black)
  - o Allow unspent funds from employees' FSAs or HRAs to be rolled over to their HSAs – H.R. 1175 (Paulsen)
  - o Allow Medicare enrollees to contribute their own money to their Medicare MSAs. – H.R. 1072 (Sanford), H.R. 1175 (Paulsen)

- Bills that Would Allow HSA Funds to Be Used for Additional Health-Related Expenses
  - o Repeal the prescription requirement for reimbursement of OTC medicines from HSAs – H.R. 247 (Brat), H.R. 394 (Jenkins), H.R. 421 (Love), H.R. 1072 (Sanford), H.R. 1175 (Paulsen), H.R. 1436 (Jordan), H.R. 1628 (Black)
  - o Allow HSA funds to be used tax-free to pay for eligible medical expenses incurred by all children under age 27 regardless of tax dependent status – H.R. 1175 (Paulsen), H.R. 5138 (Kelly)
  - Allow HSA funds to be used tax-free to pay for:
    - o insurance premiums – H.R. 247 (Brat), H.R. 408 (King), H.R. 1072 (Sanford), H.R. 1175 (Paulsen)
    - o direct primary care services or fees – H.R. 247 (Brat), H.R. 365 (Paulsen), H.R. 1072 (Sanford), H.R. 1175 (Paulsen), H.R. 1280 (Fortenberry)
    - o dietary and nutritional supplements. – H.R. 1072 (Sanford), H.R. 1175 (Paulsen)
    - o fitness and exercise equipment or health coaching, including weight loss programs. – H.R. 1072 (Sanford), H.R. 1175 (Paulsen), H.R. 1280 (Fortenberry)
    - o qualified sports and fitness expenses up to $1,000 per year ($2,000 for married couples) – H.R. 1267 (Smith), H.R. 5138 (Kelly)
  - Lower the tax penalty for non-qualified HSA distributions from 20% back to the original 10% – H.R. 247 (Brat), H.R. 1175 (Paulsen), H.R. 1436 (Jordan), H.R. 1628 (Black)
  - Allow HSA-eligible expenses incurred before the date the HSA is established to be reimbursed tax-free if the HSA account is established within 60 days of the date that the account owner's HSA-qualified coverage begins – H.R. 1175 (Paulsen), H.R. 1628 (Black)
  - Allow qualified expenses incurred prior to the date the HSA is established to be reimbursed tax-free from an HSA as long as

the account is established prior to the tax filing deadline for the year the account is established – H.R. 1072 (Sanford)

- Allow unspent FSA or HRA balances to be rolled over into an HSA as long as the amount does not exceed $2,250 for an individual with self-only coverage or $4,500 for an individual with family coverage (amounts adjusted annually for inflation); also eliminates the testing period that follows any rollover – H.R. 5138 (Kelly)

- Bills that Would Place New Restrictions on Tax-Free Uses of HSA Funds
  - Exclude elective abortions (except in the case of rape or incest) from tax-free reimbursement with HSA funds – H.R. 2019 (Foxx)
- Bills that Would Allow HSA Assets to Be Transferred/Rolled Over Tax-Free to Family Members
  - Allow an account holder's HSA to roll over to a child, parent, or grandparent, in addition to a spouse upon the account owner's death – H.R. 1072 (Sanford)
  - Allow required minimum distributions from retirement accounts to be deposited into HSAs – H.R. 277 (Roe)
- Bills that Would Protect HSA Assets from Creditors in Personal Bankruptcy Situations
  - Amend federal bankruptcy law to protect HSA assets from creditors in bankruptcy situations just as IRA assets are protected – H.R. 35 (Burgess), H.R. 1072 (Sanford), H.R. 1175 (Paulsen)
- Bills that Would Make Other HSA Changes
  - Rename "high deductible health plans" as "HSA-qualified health plans" – H.R. 1175 (Paulsen)

Chairman Roskam. Thank you.

Mr. Eyles.

STATEMENT OF MATT EYLES, PRESIDENT AND CEO, AMERICA'S INSURANCE HEALTH PLANS (AHIP)

Mr. Eyles. Chairman Roskam, Congressman Thompson, and members of the subcommittee, I am Matt Eyles, President and CEO of America's Health Insurance Plans. I appreciate this opportunity to testify on consumer-driven health plans and their role in providing Americans with access to high quality, affordable healthcare coverage.

Many AHIP members offer health insurance coverage that can be combined with health savings accounts. This is one of many options that health insurance providers offer to give consumers better choice, control, and affordability.

Millions of Americans have found this innovative combination of a tax-free savings account with insurance coverage to be an appealing option for meeting their healthcare needs.

Our written testimony focuses on three main areas.

First, some background information on HSAs, including the findings of an annual AHIP survey that has measured strong enrollment growth in HSA-eligible plans over the past 12 years, measuring over 2,000 percent increase in enrollment over this period.

Second, key issues for policymakers to consider while examining the current status and future role of HSAs and HSA eligible plans.

And third, some proposals to strengthen and improve HSA and HSA-eligible plans to better empower consumers to meet their personal needs.

Since 2005, AHIP has conducted an annual survey on enrollment in HSA-eligible plans. Our most recent survey, from April 2018, shows that enrollment in HSA-eligible plans totaled nearly 22 million as of January 2017, more than a 9 percent increase over the previous year. For context, there are now more Americans currently enrolled in HSA-eligible plans than in the entire Medicare Advantage program.

The dramatic growth in enrollment is because of the real value that HSA plans deliver: consumer choice, patient control, and the opportunity for individuals to use tax-free funds to pay current medical expenses while also setting aside money for future healthcare costs.

According to our survey results, the vast majority of HSA-eligible plans offer consumers the tools and technology to enable them to make informed decisions and spend their healthcare dollars wisely. Across markets, these resources are imperative to ensure that those enrolled in HSA-eligible plans are informed about the best way to use their funds to meet their current and future needs.

Tens of millions of consumers know the value that HSAs deliver every day, but we also know there is room for improvement. Since their enactment, there have been few changes to HSAs even as other areas of the healthcare system have experienced vast transformation, as we have learned lessons from the utilization of these accounts that has grown.

This includes a revolution in healthcare technology, a shift from volume-based to value-based payments, and a growing recognition that covering high-value services can help reduce long-term costs and improve outcomes. At the same time, healthcare costs have grown substantially for health services and treatments, especially prescription drugs, making it even more imperative that consumers have more choices and more control over their healthcare dollars.

Our testimony outlines a few solutions to make both HSAs and HSA-eligible plans even more effective and valuable options. These solutions focus broadly on three priorities.

Number one, allowing greater benefit design flexibility for HSA-eligible plans. Specifically, HSA-eligible plans should be allowed to provide pre-deductible coverage for services that help Americans manage their chronic conditions just as they do for preventive care. This would improve the value of HSA-eligible plans for consumers and enable patients to more easily access care they need to effectively manage their health, potentially avoiding debilitating and costly complications.

Number two, increasing flexibility for HSA contributions and how these funds are used. The maximum HSA contribution limit should be increased to align with the maximum out-of-pocket expenditure limits that apply to HSA-eligible plans. We believe the consumer should also be allowed to use HSA funds to easily pay for over-the-counter drugs and services and products that improve health, such as telemedicine consultations and other supplemental benefits.

Third and finally, improving healthcare affordability, it is critical, particularly for the middle class and self-employed, and to allow more consumers to fully utilize consumer-directed health products.

This can be accomplished in a few ways. These include aligning the out-of-pocket thresholds with actuarial value metal levels for consumer-directed plans in the individual and small group markets; clearly indicating HSA eligibility for exchange policies; allowing adult dependents to use HSAs; promoting HSA literacy; and finally, building off recent successes in the States by exploring novel ways to increase access to consumer-directed health products.

Thank you for the opportunity to discuss the value of HSAs and HSA-eligible plans. Like you, we are committed to strengthening, supporting, and improving this important and increasingly popular healthcare option. We look forward to working with you to advance solutions to deliver affordable access to high-quality coverage and care for every American.

Thank you.

"LOWERING COSTS AND EXPANDING ACCESS TO HEALTH CARE THROUGH CONSUMER-DIRECTED HEALTH PLANS," BY MATT EYLES, PRESIDENT AND CEO, AMERICA'S HEALTH INSURANCE PLANS FOR THE HOUSE WAYS AND MEANS COMMITTEE SUBCOMMITTEE ON HEALTH, JUNE 6, 2018

Chairman Roskam, Ranking Member Levin and members of the subcommittee, I am Matt Eyles, President and CEO of America's Health Insurance Plans (AHIP). AHIP is the national association whose members provide coverage for health care and related services to millions of

Americans every day. Through these offerings, we improve and protect the health and financial security of consumers, families, businesses, communities, and the nation. We are committed to market-based solutions and public-private partnerships that improve affordability, value, access, and well-being for consumers.

We appreciate the opportunity to testify on consumer-driven health plans and their role in providing more Americans with access to high quality, affordable health care coverage. The innovative products offered by AHIP's members include high-deductible health plans (HDHPs) that can be combined with Health Savings Accounts (HSAs). A growing number of Americans rely on HSA/HDHPs as a valuable health care coverage option.

Our statement focuses on the following areas:

- Background information on Health Savings Accounts (HSAs), including the findings of an annual AHIP survey that has measured strong enrollment growth in HSA-eligible plans over the past 12 years;
- Issues for policymakers to consider while examining the current status and future role of HSA/HDHPs; and
- Proposed solutions for strengthening and improving HSAs and HSA-eligible health plans to better empower consumers and meet their needs.

Background Information and AHIP Survey Findings on the Growing Popularity of HSA/HDHPs

HSAs provide an opportunity for individuals to use tax-free funds to pay current medical expenses while also setting aside money for future health care costs. These accounts offer additional tools to help consumers make affordable health care choices and control their health care dollars.

With HSAs, consumers play an active role in deciding when and how much to contribute to their accounts, how to invest in their accounts, and how to use their health dollars. The funds that individuals withdraw from their HSAs to pay for their health care services and products are not taxed. At the end of the year, any unspent dollars in an HSA can stay in the account and be used to pay for medical expenses in future years. Interest and other earnings on HSA funds accumulate in the fund and are also tax-free. This empowers consumers to make more engaged decisions about their health care while accumulating savings to pay for future health care needs.

HSAs must be combined with an HDHP, which also must meet specific requirements for deductibles and out-of-pocket expenses. For calendar year 2018, an HDHP is defined as a health plan with an annual deductible that is not less than $1,350 for self-only coverage or $2,700 for family coverage and annual out-of-pocket expenses (deductibles, co-payments, and other amounts, excluding premiums) that do not exceed $6,650 for self-only coverage or $13,300 for family coverage.

Federal law specifically provides that certain preventive care services must be covered by HSA- compatible health plans prior to the deductible being met at zero cost sharing. That means that HDHP enrollees have "first dollar coverage" for a wide range of preventive health care services, including annual physical exams, screening services, immunizations, tobacco cessation programs, and routine prenatal and well-child care.

A significant number of Americans have found HSA/HDHPs to be an appealing option for meeting their health care coverage and treatment needs. Since HSAs were originally authorized by Congress in December 2003,[11] there has been a steady and significant increase in the number of Americans enrolled in HSA-eligible plans.

In April 2018, AHIP released an update to our annual survey showing that enrollment in HSA/HDHPs totaled at least 21.8 million as of January 2017, reflecting a 9.2 percent increase since the previous year.[12] This survey was based on responses from 52 insurance companies. For context,

---

[11] Medicare Prescription Drug, Improvement, and Modernization Act of 2003, Public Law 108-173.

[12] *Health Savings Accounts and High Deductible Health Plans Grow as Valuable Financial Planning Tools,* AHIP, April 2018. https://www.ahip.org/wp-content/uploads/2018/04/HSA_Report_4.12.18.pdf.

based on these and other survey results, more individuals are enrolled in HSA/HDHPs than the entire Medicare Advantage program.

AHIP has conducted an annual HSA/HDHP survey since 2005. The chart below shows that HSA/HDHP enrollment has increased at a steady, robust pace – a cumulative 2,014 percent increase – over the past 12 years. The popularity of these options is also supported by other research, which have shown even higher enrollment in HSA-eligible plans – ranging from 22 million to 31.7 million people or around 12 percent of the non-Medicare population.[13,14]

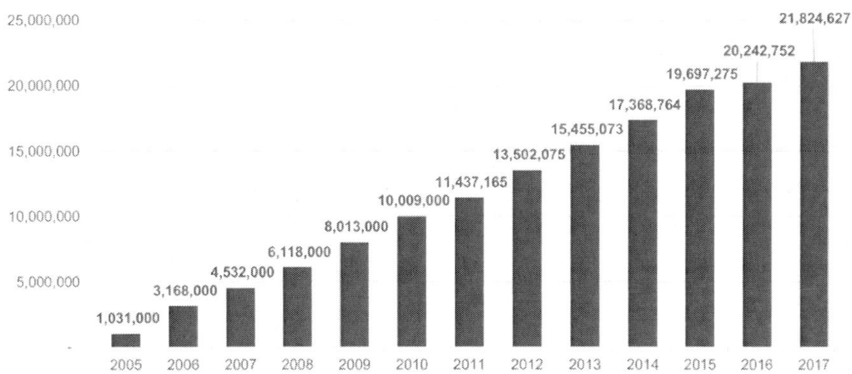

Figure 5. HSA-Qualified High-Deductible Health Plan Enrollment, 2005-2017.

Our survey also provides data on where individuals access or purchase their HSA/HDHPs and the age distribution of HSA/HDHP enrollees. These data point to other possible areas of reform, particularly for HSAs accessed on the individual and small group markets and for adults who are eligible for coverage on their parents' employer-sponsored coverage.

Demographic data for HSA/HDHP enrollees, based on AHIP's survey, show that in January 2017:

---

[13] *2017 Year-End Devenir HSA Research Report*, Devenir, February 2018. http://www.devenir.com/research/2017-year-end-devenir-hsa-research-report/.

[14] *Health Insurance Coverage: Early Release of Estimates From the National Health Interview Survey, 2017*; National Center for Health Statistics, May 2018. https://www.cdc.gov/nchs/data/nhis/earlyrelease/insur201805.pdf.

- 23 percent were under the age of 18;
- 11 percent were 18-24 years;
- 32 percent were 25-44 years;
- 33 percent were 45-64 years; and
- 1 percent were age 65 and older.

HSAs are a consumer-friendly savings tool that empowers individuals to plan for future health care expenses and gain peace of mind to supplement the security of a health insurance plan. As such, another component of our survey asked sponsors of HSA-eligible plans about the many valuable tools and services they offer to their enrollees.

We found that HDHPs offer consumers a variety of tools, including:

- 98 percent of respondents offer members access to health and wellness resources;
- 88 percent provide members access to information on their health savings account;
- 82 percent offer health care cost information;
- 69 percent supply members with access to their personal health record;
- 69 percent provide physician-specific quality data and 77 percent provide hospital-specific quality data; and
- 64 percent offer enrollees access to broker consultations.

Evidence clearly shows that HSAs have enjoyed consistent and significant growth since they were first offered to consumers in 2005. They provide an attractive option for employers, employees, and individuals seeking an efficient way to cover health care costs. There is still room for improvement to maximize the potential for consumer-directed health plans, however.

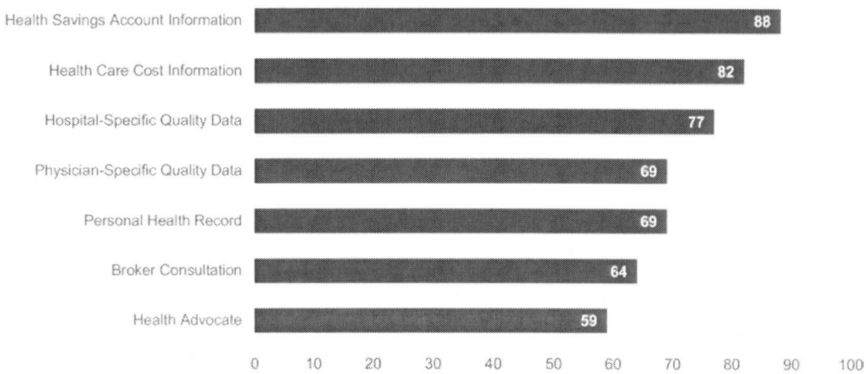

Figure 6. Percentage of Health Insurers Providing Access to Consumer Decision-Support Tools, January 2017.

Issues for Policymakers to Consider While Examining HSAs and HDHPs

As Congress evaluates the current status and future role of HSAs, it is important to look broadly at the landscape surrounding HSA/HDHPs – focusing not only on the significant value they offer consumers, but also on areas where there are opportunities for improvement.

Following the enactment of the 2003 law, there have been few changes to HSAs, even as other areas of the health care system have experienced vast transformation. These areas include a stronger emphasis on consumer agency and focus, a revolution in health technology, a shift from volume-based to value-based payments, and a growing recognition that covering high-value services can help reduce long-term costs. At the same time, costs have grown substantially for health services and treatments, making it even more imperative that consumers have adequate tools to access needed care and know their options. Policymakers must account for growing consumer reliance on these plans and their current and future health needs when considering reforms to expand flexibility for consumers, employers, and plans in their use and design of HSA/HDHPs.

Inherent Differences between the Individual Market and Group Markets Should Be Considered as Congress Explores Strategies for Strengthening HSA/HDHPs

HSA-eligible plans are available to individual market consumers, but are purchased far less frequently by individuals who buy coverage on their own than by employees who obtain coverage through group markets. Today, only about 7 percent of individuals enrolled in HSA-eligible plans are covered through the individual market. By contrast, 82 percent of enrollees in HSA-eligible plans are covered through the large group market.[15] AHIP survey data have shown that while overall enrollment in HSA/HDHPs has grown in all markets since 2005, the vast majority of growth has been concentrated in the large group market. This indicates that there are disparities in the advantages of these plans between the markets that need to be addressed to provide consumers with more cost-effective coverage options that meet consumer needs.

Employer-provided plans have distinct advantages in offering HSA-eligible plans and encouraging the use of HSAs. The most significant advantage that HSA participants have through employer-provided coverage is that most employers make direct contributions to their accounts. All contributions by an employer must be equal for all employees, regardless of income level. Thus, even for lower-wage workers who may otherwise have difficulty saving for future expenses, they will have funds in the HSA. This is a significant difference compared to the individual market, where funding the account is entirely the responsibility of the individual.

Data have shown that employers contribute significant funds to HSAs, highlighting the value they and their employees find in the accounts. For example, the Kaiser Family Foundation found that approximately 77 percent of HSA enrollees work for a firm that makes annual contributions to the HSA account.[16] The average employer contribution to the account is

---

[15] *Health Savings Accounts and High Deductible Health Plans Grow as Valuable Financial Planning Tools,* AHIP, April 2018. https://www.ahip.org/wp-content/uploads/2018/04/HSA_Report_4.12.18.pdf.

[16] *Employer Health Benefits: 2017 Annual Survey*, Kaiser Family Foundation, 2017. http://files.kff.org/attachment/Report-Employer-Health-Benefits-Annual-Survey-2017.

$608 for single coverage and $1,086 for family coverage. However, these averages include firms that contribute $0 to the account. When such firms are removed from the equation, the average contribution is $795 for single coverage and $1,417 for family coverage.

HSAs offered through employer-provided coverage also offer the advantage of providing easier access to resources to advise employees about the benefits and uses of an HSA as well as the potential to use direct payroll deductions for HSA contributions, which make it substantially easier for workers to save money, much as they do for a retirement account.

While the large group market is able to offer additional benefits that make HSA/HDHPs more attractive and practical to consumers compared to the individual and small group markets, these plans still provide an attractive option for many consumers, particularly those that may not have access to other health coverage tax advantages.

While moderate-income individuals and families have access to subsidies that shield them from premium instability in the individual market, millions of middle class Americans are increasingly being priced out of many markets. Expanding flexibility for benefit design and access to HSA-eligible plans can help increase tax-preferred access to health coverage and care for middle class individuals and families.

Currently, it is very difficult to determine whether an individual enrolled in a plan in the individual market is also eligible to enroll in an HSA. As we previously noted, the Internal Revenue Service sets out-of-pocket limits on HDHPs, which are $6,650 for self-only coverage or $13,300 for family coverage for 2018. Any health plan that has out-of-pocket limits above these thresholds cannot be coupled with an HSA. These requirements are not aligned with current metal level plan requirements, however. For example, out-of-pocket limits for individual Silver-level plans (historically the most popular coverage option) are $7,150 for individuals and $14,300 for families for 2018. Because of the misalignment in thresholds, individuals enrolled in these polices may not have access to tax-preferred mechanisms that can help cover these out-of-pocket costs.

Additionally, it is not readily apparent on HealthCare.gov which plans are and are not compatible with HSAs.

Patients with Chronic Conditions Face Barriers due to Restrictions on HSA-Eligible Plans

While HSA/HDHPs meet many consumer needs, they are generally considered a less attractive option for consumers with known, ongoing health needs – generally known as chronic conditions. Chronic diseases affect millions of Americans and are a leading driver of rising health costs. At least 60 percent of Americans live with a chronic disease, with at least 42 percent having multiple chronic conditions.[17] Moreover, 86 percent of total health care expenditures are for individuals living with chronic health conditions, accounting for $2.3 trillion annually. In recent years, there has been a growing recognition that lowering financial barriers to essential, high-value services – for example, through value-based insurance design (VBID) – can lead to better patient adherence to treatment, better clinical outcomes, and lower costs from avoiding preventable complications.

Unfortunately, federal law has not evolved to address the needs of the growing number of consumers with chronic conditions who may be enrolled in HSA/HDHPs or may want to enroll in these plans if they provided more benefit flexibility. As stated previously, HSA-eligible plans cover certain preventive services pre-deductible with no cost sharing – just like other comprehensive plans (e.g., HMO and PPO plans). However, current law takes a limited view of "preventive services" and places strict limits on what HSA-eligible plans may cover on a pre-deductible basis.

For example, this means that a diabetic enrolled in an HDHP will have to meet the plan deductible before the plan can cover insulin or test strips even though there is ample evidence showing this type of secondary and tertiary prevention is critical to avoiding debilitating, expensive complications.[18] Many consumers with chronic conditions or who have

---

[17] *Multiple Chronic Conditions in the United States*, Christine Buttorff, Teague Ruder, and Melissa Bauman, RAND Corporation, May 2017. https://www.rand.org/content/dam/rand/pubs/tools/TL200/TL221/RAND_TL221.pdf.

[18] *Primary, secondary, and tertiary prevention of non-insulin-dependent diabetes,* A. Dornhorst and P. K. Merrin. https://www.ncbi.nlm.nih.gov/pmc/articles/PMC2397691/?page=1.

dependents with chronic conditions may find it challenging to rely on an HDHP for these reasons.

Narrow Definitions Prevent Individuals from Realizing the Full Potential of HSA/HDHPs

A range of popular and cost-effective services disqualify a health plan from HSA-eligibility, if the plan offers them on a first-dollar coverage or pre-deductible basis. These services include telemedicine, second-opinion services, retail clinics, and on-site medical clinics. While many plans lower or eliminate co-pays for these services as a way of encouraging lower-cost, effective care, current federal regulations disqualify these plans from being paired with an HSA.

Similarly, HSAs cannot be used to pay for certain expenses and products that help support health and financial security. For example, an individual may not use HSA funds to pay for over-the- counter drugs that often cost less than prescription medications. HSA funds also may not be used to pay for coverage that positively impacts physical, mental, and financial health such as dental insurance, disability income protection, supplemental health benefits, Medigap coverage, and vision insurance.

While an HSA may be used to pay for Qualified Long-Term Care Insurance (QLTCI), current HSA contribution limits are often too restrictive to allow for QLTCI purchases. This is a significant concern, considering that the Department of Health and Human Services (HHS) estimates that individuals and their families pay for 52 percent of their long-term care costs out of their own pockets.[19]

The Value of HSAs Is Restrained by Statutory Limits on HSA Contributions

Statutory limits on HSA contributions limit the ability of consumers to save for their deductible and future health care expenses. For 2018, the law

---

[19] *Long-Term Services and Supports for Older Americans: Risks and Financing Research Brief,* Office of the Assistant Secretary for Planning and Evaluation, Department of Health and Human Services, July 1, 2015. https://aspe.hhs.gov/basic-report/long-term-services-and-supports-older-americans-risks-and-financing-research-brief.

limits HSA contributions to $3,450 for individual coverage and $6,900 for family coverage. However, the maximum out-of-pocket expenditure for an HSA-eligible plan is $6,650 for individual coverage and $13,300 for family coverage.

This leaves a significant gap between the annual contribution limit and the maximum-out-of-pocket limit, meaning that an individual or family may have a maximum out-of-pocket amount or deductible amount that is nearly double the amount they may save in their HSA for any given year. Thus, an account intended to provide tax-advantaged funds to help cover out-of-pocket health care expenses cannot, under current law, adequately cover the actual costs a consumer may incur in a calendar year under their specific plan.

Moreover, if an individual has an HSA but no longer has HDHP coverage, he or she cannot contribute additional amounts to the HSA under current law. This restricts a person's ability to continue to save for future expenses, including expensive medications, Medicare premiums, and long-term care.

As a direct result of the current limitations on HSA contributions, many consumers are unable to save enough money for future health care expenses, including the costs they will face in retirement, which are estimated to total $280,000 for the average couple.[20]

Given these and other restrictions on benefit design and coverage, there are 44.5 million individuals enrolled in HDHPs whose plans fail to qualify for an HSA.[21]

---

[20] *Fidelity Investments' 16th annual retiree health care cost estimate*, Fidelity Investments, April 19, 2018. https://www.fidelity.com/about-fidelity/employer-services/a-couple-retiring-in-2018-would-need-estimated-280000.

[21] *Health Insurance Coverage: Early Release of Estimates from the National Health Interview Survey, 2017*; National Center for Health Statistics, May 2018. https://www.cdc.gov/nchs/data/nhis/earlyrelease/insur201805.pdf.

Valuable Lessons on Improving HSAs and HSA-Eligible Plans Can Be Learned from Both Medicaid and the Employer Markets

States operating under a federal Medicaid waiver have experimented with HSAs for Medicaid enrollees and demonstrated that low-income individuals can effectively use HSAs and have an impact on an enrollee's utilization of health care services.

For example, the Healthy Indiana Plan (HIP) 2.0 pairs an HDHP with an HSA product called a Personal Wellness and Responsibility (POWER) Account. Under the HIP Plus version of this program, beneficiaries must contribute to a personal account. More than 90 percent of these beneficiaries consistently contributed to their POWER accounts. Rates of non-urgent emergency room visits declined for the HIP Plus population, and they used more preventive care than those in a regular HIP plan that did not contribute to a POWER account.[22] This outcome offers helpful lessons on how consumer decision-making is affected by an individual's participation in contributing funds to their HSAs.

For states and health insurers alike, the lessons from Medicaid Managed Care plans are highly instructive in designing plans for individual market consumers that may be more constrained in their ability to contribute to an HSA. More novel approaches can aid the ability of consumers to save through an HSA while also harnessing the positive results of consumer engagement through consumer-driven health products.

Proposed Solutions for Building on the Success of HSAs and HDHPs

We thank committee members for supporting innovative policy solutions to strengthen and improve HSA/HDHPs. Americans value a consumer-oriented approach to making decisions about their health care

---

[22] *Health savings accounts in the individual market*, Deloitte, 2017. https://www2.deloitte.com/content/dam/Deloitte/us/Documents/life-sciences-health-care/us-lshc-health-savings-accounts-in-the-individual-market.pdf.

needs. The enormous growth in enrollment in HSA/HDHPs clearly signals growing popularity and reliance on these plan options. This continued increase in enrollment combined with health trends and current restrictions, mean that while these plans satisfy many consumer needs, more changes are warranted to empower consumers and support Americans' physical, mental, and financial health and stability. Below, we outline several policies that would make HSA/HDHPs an even more effective and valuable health care option for the American people, many of which are championed by members of this committee.

Allow Greater Benefit Design Flexibility for HSA-Eligible Plans

As previously discussed, an enrollee in an HSA-qualified plan must meet his or her full deductible before the plan can pay for most services, treatments, or medications. Recognizing that preventive treatment is critical to improving health outcomes and avoiding costly long-term complications, Congress allowed for preventive care to be covered pre-deductible. There is a similar recognition that ensuring consistent access to treatment for those with chronic conditions such as diabetes, heart disease, and substance use disorders can help prevent expensive, debilitating complications.

The Chronic Disease Management Act (H.R. 4978) would provide much-needed flexibility by allowing HSA-qualified plans to cover services that help Americans manage their chronic conditions pre-deductible just as they do for preventive care. This approach improves the value of HSA-qualified plans for consumers and enables patients to more easily access care they need to effectively manage their chronic conditions.

Increase Flexibility for HSA Contributions and Use

HSAs are a valuable tool for consumers to use tax-free dollars for current and future health needs, but added flexibility on how these dollars are contributed would improve their utility for consumers.

Current limits for HSA contributions are not aligned with potential out-of-pocket costs for consumers, limiting the effectiveness and promise of these accounts, which are intended to help consumers better afford present and future medical costs. Policymakers should better align current contribution limits with potential out-of-pocket costs in HDHPs.

AHIP data also show that for the non-Medicare population, individuals aged 18-24 are the least likely to enroll in an HSA/HDHP even though this demographic would logically be well-suited to a plan with lower expected annual health costs and the ability to save funds for future health needs.

Unfortunately, the HSA law has not accommodated other changes to insurance coverage. While adults are now able to maintain coverage through their parents' employer-sponsored insurance up until age 26, individuals cannot contribute to or use HSA funds for adult children.

Additionally, individuals are limited in how they can use their HSA funds even for products and services that are critical to the long-term health, quality of life, and financial stability for most Americans such as dental and vision coverage, other supplemental benefits, and over-the-counter medications. Such products and services should qualify as HSA-eligible medical expenses.

Among other policies, the Bipartisan HSA Improvement Act (H.R. 5138), the Restoring Access to Medication Act (H.R. 394), and the Health Savings Act of 2017 (H.R. 35/H.R. 1175) would all allow for many of these new flexibilities.

Improve Health Care Affordability, Particularly for Middle Class Consumers and the Self- Employed, to Allow More Consumers to Fully Utilize Consumer-Directed Health Products

Millions of middle-class Americans who have annual incomes above 400 percent of the federal poverty level, but lack access to employer-provided coverage or public programs, find health insurance premiums to be unaffordable due to instability in individual market premiums. While the states and Congress have enacted policies to reduce premiums such as reinsurance funding and temporary relief from the Health Insurance Tax, more is needed.

A significant number of those who purchase health coverage through the individual marketplaces are self-employed. In fact, one in five who purchased coverage during the first year of the ACA marketplaces were either small business owners or self-employed.[23] These individuals need access to more affordable coverage. Improvements to HSAs may offer new tax advantages and more ways to save money for the self-employed and middle-class consumers.

Aligning thresholds in the individual market, clearly indicating HSA-eligibility for individual market policies, and promoting HSA literacy would improve the ability of middle-class families to choose a health plan that meets their needs and increases access to tax-preferred health coverage mechanisms.

Additionally, policymakers on both the state and federal level should build off of recent successes in many states and explore novel ways to increase access to consumer-driven health products for lower and moderate-income individuals and families.

Conclusion

With more than 21.8 million consumers covered in HSA-eligible plans, and enrollment expected to continue growing in the coming years, HSAs and HSA-eligible plans represent a vital option to provide Americans with greater control and choice over their health and financial security. Promoting consumer and patient choice in the health care system is important to improving health outcomes and patient satisfaction. HSA-eligible plans are one option among many that health plans strive to offer to provide choice and affordability for consumers.

Thank you for this opportunity to discuss the value of HSA/HDHPs and our recommendations for further strengthening and improving this important and increasingly popular health care option.

---

[23] *The Rise of Alternative Work Arrangements: Evidence and Implications for Tax Filing and Benefit Coverage*, Office of Tax Analysis Working Paper 114, Department of the Treasury, January 2017. https://www.treasury.gov/resource-center/tax-policy/tax-analysis/Documents/WP-114.pdf.

Recognizing that a growing number of Americans are embracing a consumer-oriented approach to health care, we fully support efforts in Congress to build upon the success of HSA/HDHPs.

We appreciate the support many committee members have demonstrated for HSA/HDHPs and we look forward to continuing to work with you to advance solutions for improving access to high quality, affordable health care.

Chairman Roskam. Thank you.

Ms. Dietel.

STATEMENT OF JODY DIETEL, CHIEF COMPLIANCE OFFICER, WAGEWORKS, INC.

Ms. Dietel. Thank you, Chairman Roskam, Ranking Member Levin, and members of the subcommittee. My name is Jody Dietel, and I am the chief compliance officer for WageWorks, Inc., a leading provider of consumer-directed benefit accounts, including health savings accounts, health reimbursement arrangements, and health flexible spending accounts.

WageWorks administers consumer-directed plans for about 85,000 employers across the Nation, including the FSAFeds program. Our services cover more than 7 million employees, most of whom participate in a health FSA or health savings account.

Due to the nature of our administrative services and our diverse client base, we have access to significant and compelling data, which we monitor and analyze on a regular basis to help improve our services.

Let me share some highlights of our data with you.

Many people assume that HSAs are used primarily by highly paid employees. Our data shows this to be incorrect. The median household income for an HSA account holder in our book of business is $56,100. It has rapidly declined over the last few years as HSAs have become far more prevalent.

Additionally, nearly 77 percent of those contributing to HSAs in our book of business were born after 1965, belonging to the Gen Z, millennial, and Gen X demographic. Only about 22 percent of our participants are baby boomers.

People also assume that individuals stuff large amounts of moneys into their HSAs; however, our data shows consistent average annual contributions over time, ranging from a low of just over $1,000 in 2010 to a high of $1,500 in 2017. With annual statutory contribution limits ranging from $2,900 to $6,760, depending on coverage level, this contribution data defies the notion that employees are using HSAs for means other than funding their medical expenses.

In fact, HSA account holders in our book are largely spending their fund balances. Our data shows that over the last 7 years, amounts ranging from just 25 to 35 percent of annual contributions are carried into the next year for future out-of-pocket expenses.

Sixty-six percent of transactions and nearly 70 percent of spending is on inpatient and outpatient medical care, and 33 percent of the transactions and about 13 percent of dollars spent are spent on prescription drugs.

As members of this committee know, employers are faced with increasing health plan design challenges in their quest to contain costs while maintaining a healthy and productive workforce.

One example of an unnecessary hurdle is the existing HSA eligibility rules. These limit employers' ability to offer value-based insurance designs, which can help pay for specified chronic disease services necessary to improve treatment adherence and condition management.

Employers are also largely prevented from offering certain telemedicine services or access to near-site or on-site clinics while also maintaining an employee's eligibility to contribute to an HSA.

Other design challenges include the ability of a working senior or an individual covered by Indian Tribal Health Services or TRICARE to contribute to an HSA.

Also, an employee whose spouse may have a health FSA is prevented from contributing to an HSA even though they are covered by a qualified high-deductible plan.

Outside data indicates that an increasing number of employers are moving to high-deductible health plans, and this trend only increases the important role of HSAs.

Another major challenge for employers is the Cadillac tax. While delayed until 2022, which we thank you for, this excise tax still looms large. As currently enacted, it appears that employee contributions to HSAs and health FSAs are included in the calculation of the tax.

To keep costs below the threshold, employers may have no other choice but to limit the amount employees may contribute to their HSA or health FSA, which ends up hurting employees who need help paying for their out-of-pocket costs. It is important to know that health FSAs are also valuable tools for working Americans because FSA funds are available on day one, rather than needing funds to accumulate before reimbursing expenses. FSAs can be designed to coordinate with health savings accounts, paying for dental and vision expenses, while allowing the HSA to pay for out-of-pocket costs. WageWorks recognizes the opportunity Congress has to enact meaningful HSA policy changes, and we would like to serve as a continued resource in that endeavor.

Thank you for inviting me here today, and I look forward to answering any questions that you may have.

Testimony before the Subcommittee on Health of the Ways and Means Committee of the House of Representatives, Hearing on Lowering Costs and Expanding Access to Health Care Consumer-Directed Health Plans, Submitted by Jody L. Dietel, ACFCI, CAS Chief Compliance Officer for WageWorks, Inc., June 6, 2018

Thank you, Chairman Roskam, Ranking Member Levin and members of the Subcommittee for the opportunity to speak with you today. My name is Jody Dietel. For the better part of the last decade, I have been the Chief Compliance Officer for WageWorks, Inc., a leading provider of consumer directed-benefit accounts, including account-based benefit plans which provide benefits in areas such as health care, child care, and commuting. In the health care arena, we provide administrative services for Health Savings Accounts (HSAs), Health Reimbursement Arrangements (HRAs) and Health Flexible Spending Accounts (Health FSAs). We appreciate the Subcommittee's interest in consumer-directed health plans as a means of lowering costs and expanding access to health coverage.

WageWorks, Inc. provides administration for nearly 85,000 employers nationwide, including the FSAFeds program offered by the Office of Personnel Management. Our services cover more than 7 million employees nationwide, the majority of whom participate in an HSA or Health FSA.

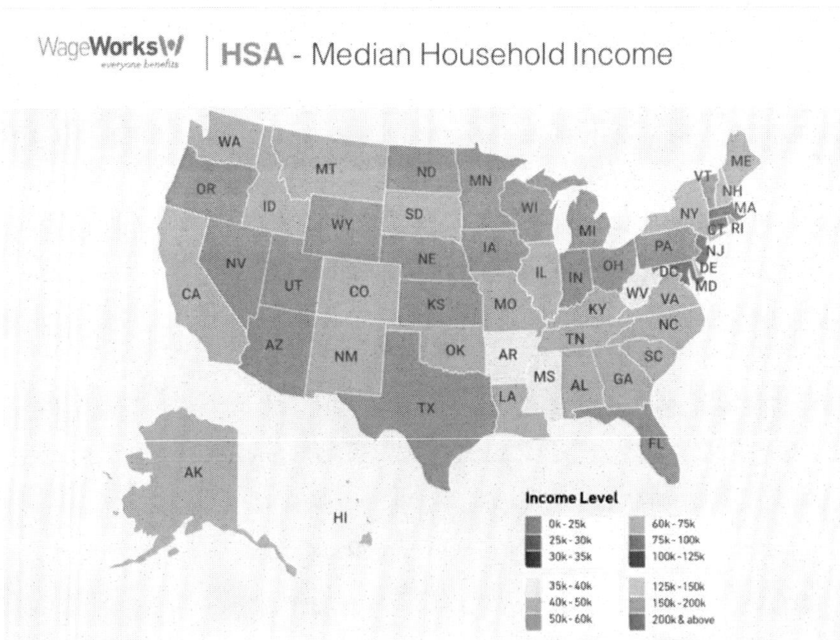

Due to the nature of our administrative services and our diverse client base, we have access to a significant amount of data which we monitor and analyze on a regular basis to help improve our services. This data provides some unique and compelling insights related to HSAs that I believe will be of interest to you as you consider ways to lower costs and expand access to these consumer-directed accounts.

An often assumed data point is that HSAs are primarily utilized by highly paid employees. Our data supports the conclusion that this assumption is incorrect. The median household income for an HSA accountholder is $57,060. In fact, HSA accountholders in just four states (Connecticut, Maryland, Massachusetts, and New Jersey) and the District of Columbia have median household incomes in excess of $75,000. In 11 other states, the median household incomes of HSA accountholders range from $60,000 to $75,000, 18 states have median household incomes ranging from $50,000 to $60,000, and in another 17 states, the median household income is less than $50,000.

WageWorks | HSA - Participation by Generation

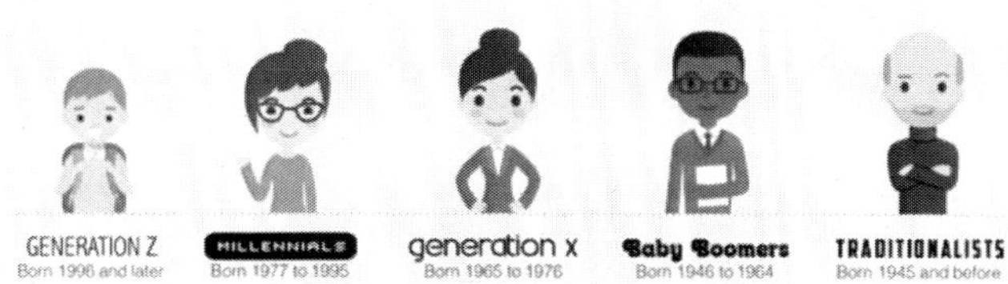
GENERATION Z
Born 1996 and later
MILLENNIALS
Born 1977 to 1995
generation x
Born 1965 to 1976
Baby Boomers
Born 1946 to 1964
TRADITIONALISTS
Born 1945 and before

Generation	Elections	Average Election	Participant Percent
Gen Z	$1,884,149	$481	0.68%
Millennials/Gen Y	$236,062,584	$846	48.44%
Gen X	$252,597,616	$1,568	27.94%
Baby Boomers	$228,262,742	$1,741	22.75%
Traditionalists	$1,241,757	$1,191	0.18%
Unknown	$7,404	$1,234	0.00%

23

Another claim we often hear is that only older workers (assumed to have more disposable income) contribute to HSAs. Our data also supports the conclusion that this too is incorrect. Specifically, we found that nearly 77% of participants contributing to an HSA were born in 1965 or after, belonging to the Gen Z, Millennial and Gen X demographic. Only about 22% of our participants are Baby Boomers.

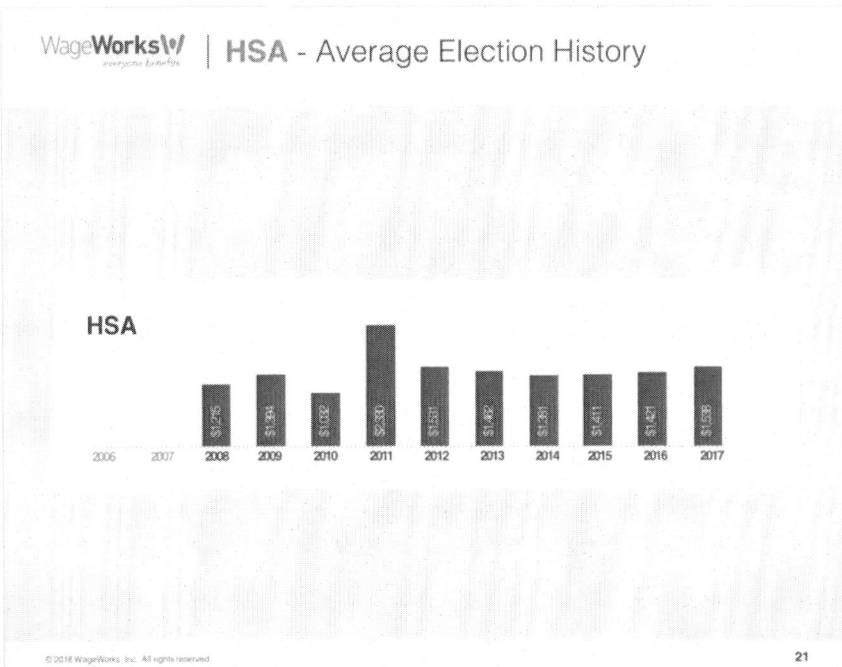

There is also an oft-stated assumption that individuals "stuff" large amounts of money into their HSAs. However, our data illustrates generally consistent average annual contributions over time, ranging from a low of $1,032 in 2010 to a high of $1,538 in 2017.[24] With annual contribution limits ranging from $2,900 to $6,760 during the same time frame (depending on whether the accountholder has single or family health

[24] 2011 may be an outlier at $2,330 due to the accelerated movement to implement High-Deductible Health Plans (HDHPs) as a response to the many of the changes enacted under the Affordable Care Act (ACA) that became effective in 2011.

coverage), this contribution data stands in opposition to the notion that employees are using HSAs for means other than funding their medical expenses.

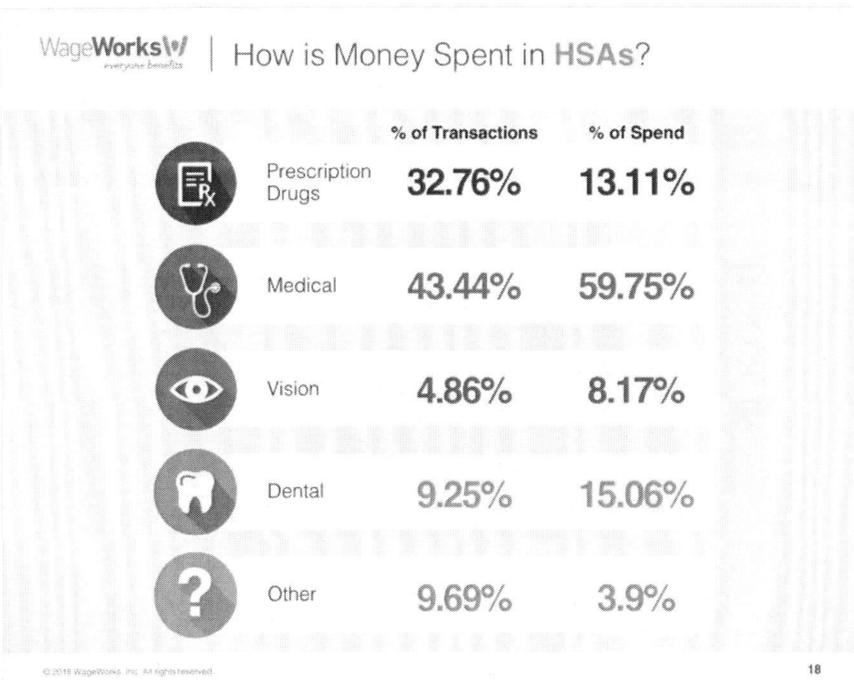
WageWorks
How is Money Spent in HSAs?
% of Transactions
% of Spend
Prescription Drugs
32.76%
13.11%
Medical
43.44%
59.75%
Vision
4.86%
8.17%
Dental
9.25%
15.06%
Other
9.69%
3.9%
18

We also analyzed the data for spending trends among the participant accounts that WageWorks administers. While it may be assumed that accountholders are using their HSA as a long-term savings vehicle, we found that accountholders are largely spending-down their balances. For example, our data shows that over the last seven years, amounts ranging from just 25% to 35% of annual contributions are carried into the next year for future out-of-pocket expenses. At the same time, we found that 66% of transactions and 69% of spending is on both inpatient and outpatient care at health care providers, while almost 33% of transactions and 13% of spending is attributed to prescription drugs.

Barriers Employers Face When Establishing Consumer-Directed Health Plans

Employers are challenged when designing health care plans to meet multiple objectives such as containing costs, maintaining a healthy and productive workforce, providing coverage tools for those with chronic conditions and providing access for employees to manage rising out-of-pocket costs. Unfortunately, many of the existing HSA rules have not kept pace with innovative design solutions that many employers want to utilize.

For example, the existing HSA eligibility rules limit an employer's ability to offer value-based insurance designs intended to help pay for specified chronic care services necessary to improve treatment adherence and condition management. Specifically, in cases where an employer wants to design an otherwise HSA-qualified High-Deductible Health Plan (HDHP) to pay for certain chronic care services before the deductible is met, this design – while advantageous to an employee with a chronic condition – will render this employee ineligible to contribute to an HSA.

Currently, HSA-qualified HDHPs are permitted to cover certain "preventive services" before the deductible is met without disqualifying HSA participation. However, coverage for "other services" is considered coverage before the deductible is met, thus disqualifying covered individuals from contributing to an HSA. These other services can include reducing or eliminating cost-sharing or deductibles for specified high-value medications and services, such as medications to control blood pressure or diabetes, and may save money by reducing future expensive medical procedures and improving the health status of the patient. Value-based insurance designs have been shown to improve adherence to medication regiments, quality measures, health outcomes, and patient experience, yet these designs adversely affect an employee's eligibility to contribute to an HSA.

Employers are also largely prohibited from offering certain telemedicine services or access to near-site/on-site clinics while also maintaining an employee's eligibility to contribute to an HSA. Such services and access in most cases are considered "coverage under the deductible" and thus disqualify employees from contributing to an HSA, even though the employee is covered under an HSA-qualified HDHP.

It is important to note that telemedicine allows patients to save transportation costs and time, provides access to care for individuals living in rural areas and other underserved locations, and also reduces the need for individuals to miss work due to doctor's appointments and other medical care. Additionally, it helps patients avoid waiting rooms where other ill patients are waiting for provider visits—thus reducing the chance of secondary illness.

Access to near-site or on-site clinics began in the 1980s, usually as a way to treat occupational injuries typically in heavy-industry or manufacturing industries. As those industries declined, so did the number of employers with on-site clinics. However, in the past 10 years or so, on-site clinics have experienced a renewed popularity as they give employers the opportunity to better control healthcare delivery costs. Additionally, many on-site clinics offer lower or no co-pays to employees. On-site clinics have been shown to improve employees' focus on preventive care, including diagnostic screenings and flu shots. The increased access to on-site clinics may reduce absenteeism because employees are less likely to work while ill or develop a more serious illness (which requires them to remain at home) due to lack of appropriate medical care.

Unfortunately, most telemedicine and near-site/on-site clinics disqualify employees from contributing to an HSA because such telemedicine services or access to near-site/on-site clinics are considered impermissible coverage below the statutorily mandated deductible for HSA-qualified HDHPs (for 2018, the minimum deductible for an HSA-qualified HDHP is $1,350 for single and $2,700 for family coverage).

Additionally, some employers are establishing direct primary care relationships, which provide primary care for a fixed fee. These arrangements are shown to improve access to preventive services, better health outcomes and provide more coordinated care for patients, often with significant cost savings. These too disqualify a participant from contributing to an HSA.

There are other eligibility requirements that are fairly rigid, preventing employees from contributing to an HSA. These include the inability for a working senior who is eligible for Medicare Part A or an individual covered by Indian Tribal Health Services or TriCare to contribute to an HSA. This inability also extends to those covered by a health care sharing ministry, which is designed as a consumer-directed option. Also, an employee whose spouse has a Health FSA is prevented from contributing to an HSA, even though this employee is covered under an HSA-qualified HDHP.

Currently, HSA accountholders who are older than age 55 can make catch-up contributions of $1,000 annually. Unfortunately, current law requires a spouse to make their catch-up contribution to a different account, which is confusing and administratively burdensome for the consumer. This is another example of "eligibility rigidity" that should and could be addressed for the purposes of removing outdated barriers to HSA adoption and use.

With the Increased Number of High-Deductible Health Plans (HDHPs), Congress Should Make It Easier to Access an HSA

Outside data indicates that an increasing number of employers are moving to HDHPs. This trend will only increase the important role played by HSAs. According to Kaiser Family Foundation's (KFF) 2017 Employer Health Benefits Survey,[25] 58% of covered workers are employed in a firm that offers more than one health plan type. Seventy percent of covered workers in large firms are employed by a firm that offers more than one plan type, compared to 30% in small firms.

About 57% of covered workers work in firms that offer one or more HDHPs with Savings Options. Among covered workers in firms offering only one type of health plan, those in large firms are more likely to be

[25] http://files.kff.org/attachment/Report-Employer-Health-Benefits-Annual-Survey-2017.

offered an HDHP with Savings Options (36%) than those in small firms (23%). Among covered workers in firms offering only one type of health plan, 30% are in firms that only offer an HDHP with Savings Options.

In recently released data from the 2017 National Health Interview Survey,[26] 43.7% of people under age 65 with private health insurance were enrolled in an HDHP, including 18.2% who were enrolled in a consumer-driven health plan (i.e., an HDHP paired with an HSA) and 25.5% who were enrolled in an HDHP without an HSA. Among those with private health insurance, enrollment in HDHPs has generally increased from 25.3% in 2010 to 43.7% in 2017.

HDHPs are attractive to both employers and employees alike as they generally have lower premium costs. Data from the KFF 2017 Employer Health Benefits Survey supports this proposition: "The average annual premiums for covered workers in an HDHP with Savings Options are lower for single coverage ($6,024) and family coverage ($17,581) than overall average premiums. The average premiums for covered workers enrolled in PPO plans are higher for single ($6,965) and family coverage ($19,481) than the overall plan average."[27] It is important to note, however, that there are wide variations in premiums based on several factors, including group size, region, industry, age demographics, wage level, union status and firm ownership. These factors and the impact on premiums are also discussed in the KFF report.

Common sense changes to address the eligibility issues discussed above would serve to make HDHPs paired with an HSA far less confusing and more workable for American workers and employers. Additionally, while average contributions are not anywhere near the maximum HSA contribution limits (as illustrated by our data, discussed above), accountholders should be able to protect themselves against the maximum out-of-pocket exposure they have, so contribution limits should be aligned with the HSA out-of-pocket limits (for 2018, the HSA out-of-pocket limits are $6,650 for single and $13,300 for family coverage). As a reference point, the Milliman Medical Index (MMI) reports out-of-pocket costs

[26] https://www.cdc.gov/nchs/data/nhis/earlyrelease/insur201805.pdf.

[27] http://files.kff.org/attachment/Report-Employer-Health-Benefits-Annual-Survey-2017.

reaching $4,704 in 2018, up from $4,534 in 2017.[28] Out-of-pocket costs are expected to continue to increase each year.

Other Challenges Employers Face

Another challenge for employers is the Cadillac Tax. While delayed until 2022, this excise tax still looms large. As currently enacted, it appears that employee contributions to HSAs and Health FSAs will be included in the calculation of the Tax. To keep costs below the thresholds, employers may have no other choice but to limit the amount employees may contribute to their HSA or Health FSA, which ends up hurting employees who need help paying for their out- of-pocket costs. A Commonwealth Fund issue brief indicates this: "Thus, at least initially, these savings accounts, rather than enrollee cost-sharing or other plan features, are likely to be affected most by the tax as employers act to limit their HSA contributions."[29] More pointedly, in response to the Cadillac Tax, the American Health Policy Institute found that about 19% of large employers were already curtailing or eliminating employee contributions to Health FSAs and about 13% of large employers were curtailing or eliminating employee contributions to HSAs.[30]

It is important to note that Health FSAs are additional tools valued by working Americans because FSA funds are available in their entirety on the first day of the year, rather than needing funds to accumulate before reimbursing expenses. In fact, based on anecdotal data from WageWorks participants—and common sense—shows that those with chronic or serious illnesses often fare better with a Health FSA than an HSA because

---

28 http://www.milliman.com/uploadedFiles/insight/Periodicals/mmi/2018-milliman-medical-index.pdf. The Milliman Medical Index (MMI) is an actuarial analysis of the projected total cost of health care for a hypothetical family of four covered by an employer-sponsored preferred provider organization (PPO) plan. Unlike many other healthcare cost reports, the MMI measures the total cost of healthcare benefits, not just the employer's share of the costs, and not just premiums.

29 http://www.commonwealthfund.org/publications/issue-briefs/2016/june/cadillac-tax.

30 http://www.americanhealthpolicy.org/Content/documents/resources/AHPI_Excise_Tax_October_2015.pdf.

their spending occurs early in the year, and the immediate availability of Health FSA elections (even though funds have not actually been contributed yet) helps participants afford their sometimes significant out-of- pocket costs. In addition, FSAs can be designed to coordinate with HSAs, paying for dental and vision expenses, while allowing the HSA to pay for out-of-pocket costs under the medical plan.

Finally, most employer plans today have high deductibles. For example, KFF's 2017 Employer Health Benefits Survey notes that 81% of covered workers are enrolled in a plan with an annual deductible, and that the average annual deductible for single coverage is $1,505,[31] which is higher than the HSA-qualified HDHP's statutory minimum deductible (e.g., for 2017, the minimum deductible for an HSA-qualified HDHP was $1,300 for single coverage). This and other design challenges often lead to confusion about whether a plan is actually an HSA-qualified plan or a just an HDHP with features that render an employee ineligible to contribute to an HSA. A simple way to resolve this confusion is by changing the law to refer to an HDHP that preserves an employee's eligibility to contribute to an HSA as an "HSA-Eligible Health Plan," which is a change that would be welcomed by the employer community.

WageWorks recognizes the opportunity Congress has to enact meaningful HSA policy changes and follows closely the various legislative proposals in both the House and Senate that will address many of the eligibility issues I have raised herein. These include changing the name of an HDHP that otherwise qualifies as an HSA-qualified HDHP to an "HSA-Eligible Health Plan," fixing the eligibility issues faced by those with "other coverage" such as Indian Tribal Health Services, TriCare, Medicare Part A, and those whose spouse may have a Health FSA and allowing employers greater freedom in plan design to include chronic care services, direct primary care, value-based coverage and telemedicine, along with access to on-site or near-site clinics. We thank the Committee on Ways and Means for all of their efforts to enact common sense HSA reforms, and we

[31] http://files.kff.org/attachment/Report-Employer-Health-Benefits-Annual-Survey-2017.

would be happy to serve as a continued resource as these proposals move through the legislative process.

Thank you for your time.

Chairman Roskam. Thank you.

Ms. Glied.

STATEMENT OF SHERRY GLIED, DEAN, NEW YORK UNIVERSITY, ROBERT F. WAGNER GRADUATE SCHOOL OF PUBLIC SERVICE

Ms. Glied. Chairman Roskam, Ranking Member Levin, and members of the subcommittee, I am Sherry Glied, professor and dean of the Robert F. Wagner Graduate School of Public Service at New York University. Thank you for inviting me to testify.

The U.S. healthcare system is in much better shape today than it was 10 years ago. The uninsurance rate has fallen by nearly half. The rate of growth of healthcare spending is at historic lows.

But there is increasing concern about maintaining the affordability of healthcare. That is because, although many more Americans are insured today, there have been changes in the nature of coverage.

High-deductible health plans not only continue to dominate the non-group health insurance market, as they always have, but they now make up nearly half the plans offered to employees.

Analyses by the Federal Reserve Board, however, show that over one-third of all American adults don't have enough income and savings to shoulder an unexpected emergency bill of just $400, well below the deductible in a high-deductible plan. That low level of financial security is on a collision course with this rise in high deductibles.

HSAs offer a tax break, that is a tax expenditure, to people who have specialized savings accounts. Relaxing the rules on HSAs would make that HSA tax break and expenditure bigger.

But would increasing those tax breaks be a good way to allocate scarce public resources toward addressing the affordability problems that are of growing concern to many Americans? A robust body of evidence says the answer is, no, relaxing HSA rules in general would not be a cost-effective way to address these concerns.

One critical reason is that there is a mismatch between those who would gain from HSA tax breaks and those who actually need the financial protection. It is lower, middle-income Americans who face real problems paying medical bills. But people with incomes in this range face very low marginal tax rates, and that means that they gain very few benefits from the tax breaks afforded to health savings accounts.

Instead, those tax breaks are most valuable to people in the highest marginal tax brackets, and in that group very few people have difficulty paying medical bills. So every extra dollar of tax expenditures devoted to HSAs buys very little gain in healthcare affordability.

As we would expect, higher-income people are more than four times as likely to open HSAs and to fully fund them than are those with lower incomes. Because of those patterns, we find that for lower, middle-income households in high-deductible plans, whether you have an HSA or not has absolutely no effect on whether you can afford to pay your medical bills.

Another problem is that we now know that the basic idea here, to encourage smarter consumption of healthcare through consumer-directed health plans, while theoretically elegant, is flawed in practice. Most people do not treat their HSAs as savings vehicles. They don't accumulate money in them.

Instead, for people who are relatively healthy and who don't anticipate using a lot of services, the tax break for HSAs effectively reduces the first-dollar cost of care. It undoes the effect of the deductible.

Expanding the scope of HSAs would just give healthy, higher-income Americans, the ones who put money into their plans, even bigger discounts on a broad range of discretionary medical services like over-the-counter drugs and prescription sunglasses.

It also turns out that having a consumer-directed plan does not make people smarter consumers. People with consumer-directed health plans spend more on expenses that aren't covered by health insurance at all, like those sunglasses, but they also use fewer preventive services and they are less likely to adhere to necessary treatment.

That holds even when the health plans explicitly and publicly exempt preventive services, like cancer screenings and vaccinations, from the deductibles.

Finally, consumers with consumer-directed health plans are not better shoppers. Study after study of consumer-directed health plans have found no evidence whatsoever that these mechanisms, including the transparency tools that go with them, lead to price shopping or to lower prices for key services like office visits and inpatient care.

That is really important because the factor that is driving up costs in the private market today is the high price of care, not excess utilization.

All in all, simply expanding HSAs and consumer-directed health plans is a costly solution in search of a problem. It won't improve affordability for those who have the most problems paying health bills, it won't improve the efficiency with which Americans use their healthcare, and it won't contribute to containing healthcare costs.

Thank you.

TESTIMONY OF SHERRY GLIED, PHD, DEAN AND PROFESSOR OF PUBLIC SERVICE, ROBERT F. WAGNER GRADUATE SCHOOL OF PUBLIC SERVICE, NEW YORK UNIVERSITY TO THE SUBCOMMITTEE ON HEALTH OF THE HOUSE WAYS AND MEANS COMMITTEE, JUNE 6, 2018

The US health care system had undergone a remarkable transformation over the past eight years. The uninsured rate in the non-elderly population, which had peaked at 18.2% in 2010, fell nearly in half, to 10.4% in 2016, a rate lower than ever previously recorded[32]. Over the same period, the rate of growth of per capita health care costs in the US was much lower than over any comparable period since 1960[33]. According to data collected by the National Center for Health Statistics (NCHS), the share of Americans in families that reported having problems paying medical bills fell steadily from 2011 to 2016[34], and that decline has been associated with a decline in the number of health-care related personal bankruptcies[35] and with declines in hospital uncompensated care costs[36].

These developments mean that Americans, as a whole, are in a much better situation with respect to healthcare costs, access, and financial protection than they were a decade ago. But problems certainly remain. One of the most important is that some people, despite holding health insurance coverage, cannot afford care when they need it. Deductibles, coinsurance rates, and exposure to out-of-pocket medical expenses have been rising rapidly. While high deductible health plans have always been quite common among those purchasing insurance in the non-group market, today, according to the NCHS, nearly half of those with employer-sponsored health insurance are in high deductible health plans (those with deductibles over $1300 for an individual or $2600 for a family). For many families, these deductibles are very large relative to income and savings. As a consequence, many Americans who hold insurance coverage are effectively underinsured[37]. They do not have the savings available to pay

---

32 https://www.kff.org/uninsured/slide/uninsured-rate-among-the-nonelderly-population-1972-2017/.

33 Author's tabulations of the National Health Expenditure Accounts. https://www.cms.gov/Research-Statistics-Data-and-Systems/Statistics-Trends-and-Reports/NationalHealthExpendData/NationalHealthAccountsHistorical.html.

34 Cohen, Robin and Emily Zammitti. Problems Paying Medical Bills Among Persons Under Age 65: Early Release of Estimates From the National Health Interview Survey, 2011–June 2017. https://www.cdc.gov/nchs/data/nhis/earlyrelease/probs_paying_medical_bills_jan_2011_jun_2017.pdf.

35 St John, A. "How the Affordable Care Act drove down personal bankruptcy." *Consumer Rep* (2017).

36 Glied, Sherry, and Adlan Jackson. "The future of the Affordable Care Act and insurance coverage." *American journal of public health* 107, no. 4 (2017): 538-540.

37 Collins, Sara R., Munira Z. Gunja, and Michelle M. Doty. "How Well Does Insurance Coverage Protect Consumers from Health Care Costs?." (2017). http://www.commonwealthfund.org/publications/issue-briefs/2017/oct/insurance-coverage-consumers- health-care-costs. Collins, Sara R., Munira Z. Gunja Michelle M. Doty, and

costs below those deductible and out-of-pocket maximum levels. The Commonwealth Fund's surveys show that only about half of Americans with incomes below 250% FPL report that they are confident they could pay for care if they became sick. Similarly, according to the Federal Reserve Board's 2016 Survey of Household Economics and Decisionmaking, about 35% of American adults do not have enough income and savings to make all their other bill payments if they were unexpectedly faced with a $400 emergency[38].

This context – one of unprecedented improvements in coverage, access, and cost- containment, but continuing problems in affordability – informs new interest in the potential role of consumer-directed health plans in the US health system. As policymakers once again consider these plans, there has been an explosion of new research in health care economics, facilitated by improved access to data on health insurance claims. This new research offers very valuable insight into whether and how consumer-directed plans can fill the gaps in coverage, access, and financial protection that remain.

Consumer-directed health plans (CDHPs) were greeted with great optimism by many health policy experts when they were first introduced. My review of these plans and of the research literature since their introduction, however, suggests that this model has not lived up to these early expectations. CDHPs have not, and are not likely to, lead to more than marginal increases in the number of people who have insurance coverage. The financial benefits of tax incentives for CDHPs have largely accrued to higher income households that already held health insurance and that already had the wherewithal to pay their out-of-pocket health care expenses. Finally, CDHPs have not been an effective strategy to rationalize the consumption of health care and to reduce inefficient spending. Expanding the scope and reach of CDHP is unlikely to make any

---

Herman K. Bhupal. "Americans' Confidence in their Ability to Pay for Health Care is Falling" (2018). http://www.commonwealthfund.org/publications/blog/2018/may/americans- confidence-paying-health-care-falling.

[38] Larrimore, Jeff, Alex Durante, Christina Park, and Anna Tranfaglia. "Report on the economic well-being of US Households in 2016." *Board of Governors of the Federal Reserve System* (May 2017).

significant dent in the cost, access, and affordability problems that currently face our healthcare system.

Consumer-Directed Health Plans

Consumer-directed health plans (CDHPs) have been encouraged in the USA since 1996, through a series of temporary tax incentives. The 2003 Medicare Prescription Drug, Improvement and Modernization Act provided a permanent tax incentive for the establishment of Health Savings Accounts (HSAs) coupled with qualified high deductible health plans (HDHPs). The combination of HSAs and HDHPs is what is generally meant by CDHPs. The promotion of CDHPs was a policy response to an economic concern that generous health insurance provides an incentive for the over-use of and lack of price shopping for health services. By extending the tax incentives that exist for health insurance premiums to out-of-pocket payments, policymakers hoped to encourage people to buy higher deductible health insurance policy and thus, neutralize some of the distortionary effects of health insurance coverage[39].

In principle, CDHPs should promote insurance coverage (through the additional tax incentive they provide), offer financial protection (through the accumulation of assets in the plans), and control costs (by encouraging consumers to shop in a cost-conscious way). In practice, however, CDHPs have fallen short of these goals.

Promoting Insurance Coverage

The favorable tax benefits offered through HSAs provides a new subsidy for health insurance coverage, which may encourage people who do not have health insurance coverage to purchase it. This effect, however, is rather small. The usefulness of HSAs as a means of expanding coverage

[39] Cogan, John F., R. Glenn Hubbard, and Daniel P. Kessler. "Making markets work: five steps to a better health care system." *Health Affairs* 24, no. 6 (2005): 1447-1457. Jack, William, and Louise Sheiner. "Welfare-improving health expenditure subsidies." *The American Economic Review* 87, no. 1 (1997): 206-221.

depends on two factors: the expected level of out-of-pocket expenditures under a high-deductible plan (because this determines the amount now exempt from tax), and marginal income tax rates. Both factors work against HSAs having a substantial impact on coverage. First, because health expenditures are highly skewed, most people spend very little on care each year, while a very small number of people each year account for most health expenditures. Because of this, the *average* amount a person might expect to spend under a high-deductible plan is quite low.

Second, most people without insurance coverage, even today after the ACA expansions, have low incomes and face low or zero marginal tax rates. Together, these two factors mean that the tax incentives for HSAs, even if further expanded, would induce very little increase in insurance coverage[40]. The benefits of HSAs accrue almost entirely to those with higher marginal tax rates who already have insurance. That is, the over $2 billion annual tax expenditures currently associated with HSAs do not induce additional coverage[41]; instead, they largely crowd-out existing private spending.

Improving Financial Protection

The CDHP model makes most sense when funds to pay for medical expenses under the HDHP are readily available within the HSA. Unfortunately, many people with HDHPs today do not have HSAs. Even where HSAs do exist, they are typically under-funded. This is not surprising -- other, similar, tax-favored savings vehicles, such as retirement accounts, are similarly underfunded, except among the highest income beneficiaries[42].

HSA contributions may be made by employees, employers or both. In calendar year 2017, just under half of employers who offered HSAs made

---

40 Remler, Dahlia K., and Sherry A. Glied. "How much more cost sharing will health savings accounts bring?." *Health Affairs* 25, no. 4 (2006): 1070-1078.

41 Lowry, Sean. "Health-Related Tax Expenditures: Overview and Analysis." *CRS Report, Congressional Research Service* (2016).

42 Burman, Leonard E., William G. Gale, Matthew Hall, and Peter R. Orszag. "Distributional effects of defined contribution plans and individual retirement arrangements." In *The Distributional Effects of Government Spending and Taxation*, pp. 69-111. Palgrave Macmillan, London, 2006.

no contribution at all to their employees' savings plans[43]. Employer contributions to HSAs, among those making contributions, averaged $795 for single coverage and $1416 for family coverage in 2016. Very few workers – just 2% – enrolled in a Health Savings Account (HSA)-qualified HDHP received an account contribution for single coverage at least equal to their deductible in 2017[44]. High-income and older tax filers are both much more likely to establish HSAs and to fully fund their HSAs; one recent study found that they did so at least four times as often as did low-income and younger filers[45].

Annual contributions by employers and employees account for virtually all of the value of HSAs. Most holders do not treat their HSAs as investment funds. Rather, they use them as an extra checking account to pay medical bills. According to research from EBRI, in 2016, just 4 percent of accounts had investments other than cash[46].

These patterns of underfunding and limited use as investment vehicles help explain why the use of HSAs has such an anemic effect on care affordability. As Table 1 shows, people with HDHPs report more trouble paying medical bills than do those with traditional insurance.

About 15% of adults 18-64 with private insurance who have HDHPs report difficulty paying medical bills, compared to just under 10% of those with traditional plans. That is to be expected – high deductibles increase financial exposure. What is more surprising is that the addition of an HSA does so little to mitigate this problem. Among those with incomes between 100-400% FPL, there is no difference at all in difficulty paying medical bills between those with an HDHP without an HSA and those who have an

[43] Claxton, G., M. Rae, M. Long, A. Damico, G. Foster, and H. Whitmore. "Employer Health Benefits 2017." (2017). http://files.kff.org/attachment/Report-Employer-Health-Benefits-Annual-Survey-2017.

[44] Claxton, G., M. Rae, M. Long, A. Damico, G. Foster, and H. Whitmore. "Employer Health Benefits 2017." (2017). http://files.kff.org/attachment/Report-Employer-Health-Benefits-Annual-Survey-2017.

[45] Helmchen, Lorens A., David W. Brown, Ithai Z. Lurie, and Anthony T. Lo Sasso. "Health savings accounts: growth concentrated among high-income households and large employers." *Health Affairs* 34, no. 9 (2015): 1594-1598.

[46] Fronstin, Paul. "Trends in Health Savings Account Balances, Contributions, Distributions, and Investments, 2011-2016: Statistics from the EBRI HSA Database." (2017). https://papers.ssrn.com/sol3/papers.cfm?abstract_id=3004723.

HSA. Among those with incomes above 400%FPL, about 11% of those with an HDHP and no HSA report difficulty paying medical bills, while about 8% of those with an HSA report such difficulties. While this is an improvement, even the latter figure is more than 50% higher than the rate among those with traditional insurance.

Table 2. Percentage Reporting Difficulty in Paying Medical Bills, Among those 18-64 with Private Insurance

		All	<100% FPL	100-<400% FPL	>400% FPL	Count
Traditional Plan		9.6%	11.7%	16.9%	5.2%	62,713,472
High Deductible Plan		15.2%	21.1%	25.4%	9.5%	42,628,838
	No HSA	16.8%	21.6%	25.3%	10.8%	25,042,184
	With HSA	12.8%	18.9%	25.8%	8.0%	15,092,756

Author's tabulations of the 2016 National Health Interview Survey.

Controlling Costs

A principle goal of CDHP is to improve the efficiency of how people use the health care system, and thereby to control costs. Economic research, however, suggests three main problems that impede the ability of CDHPs to achieve this goal: lower marginal costs than traditional plans for people with low health spending, inefficient service utilization decisions, and weak shopping behavior.

CDHPs are intended to reduce excess spending by requiring consumers to face more of the costs of their own health care decisions (skin in the game). In practice, however, the price (net of taxes) of medical care facing consumers is not always higher and may often be *lower* under an HSA compared with other types of insurance[47]. People who expect to have low health care spending are likely to see their after-tax out of pocket costs fall when they switch to an HSA, because their out-of-pocket costs will now be

[47] Buchmueller, Thomas C. "Consumer-Oriented Health Care Reform Strategies: A Review of the Evidence on Managed Competition and Consumer-Directed Health Insurance." *The Milbank Quarterly* 87.4 (2009): 820–841. *PMC*. Web. 3 June 2018; Remler, Dahlia K., and Sherry A. Glied. "How much more cost sharing will health savings accounts bring?." *Health Affairs* 25, no. 4 (2006): 1070-1078.

paid for out of tax-favored savings. The offsetting effects of the after-tax price reductions from HSAs on the utilization-reduction incentives of HDHPs may explain why some long-term studies of CDHPs find relatively modest, or even non-existent, savings effects. For example, Chen, Feldman, and Parente, long-time advocates of CDHPs, followed a sample of very large firms that had implemented these plans over a period of five years (2005-2009). They find that members enrolled in HSAs had comparable levels of spending compared to those in traditional plans, and those enrolled in related Health Reimbursement Accounts actually spent more than those enrolled in traditional accounts over time.[48]

The effect of this new, lower marginal price will be most acute for services that are not typically paid for through private insurance, but that are eligible for payment under HSA plan. For example, while relatively few private health insurance plans cover prescription sunglasses, these expenses may be paid using tax-favored dollars in an HSA. To the extent that HSA funds are used to pay for expenses that are not typically covered under health insurance, they both crowd out existing private out-of-pocket spending and reduce, rather than increase, efficiency across the health system. It is far from clear that it is economically desirable to devote valuable tax expenditures toward encouraging excess spending on discretionary health care services.

A second challenge for improving efficiency through CDHPs is that people are not well- informed about how best to use medical services or have limited understanding of their plans. Higher deductibles do often lead to lower rates of use of care, but these differences in rates of use are similar for valuable care and for care that is less valuable. This pattern has been observed in multiple studies dating back to the RAND Health Insurance Experiment of the late 1970s[49]. Similarly, a comparison of practices among patients with chronic conditions found that those in a CDHP were less likely to adhere to treatment. For patients with hypertension, dyslipidemia,

---

[48] Chen, Song, Roger Feldman, and Stephen T. Parente. "A five-year study of health expenditures among full replacement CDHPs, optional CDHPs and traditional managed care plans." *Insur. Mark. Co. Anal. Actuar. Comput* 5, no. 1 (2014): 6-16.

[49] Joseph P. Newhouse, and Rand Corporation. Insurance Experiment Group. *Free for all?: lessons from the RAND health insurance experiment*. Harvard University Press, 1993.

diabetes, and diabetes, enrollment in a CDHP reduced use of medications[50]. The overall effect of a high deductible appears to outweigh targeted exemptions aimed at encouraging effective utilization. For example, a recent study found that consumers enrolled in high deductible plans reduced the use of preventive services, even though these services are fully covered under such plans[51].

The final problem with improving efficiency through CDHPs is that these plans appear to operate almost entirely by affecting rates of utilization, but a growing volume of research indicates that the problems of the US health care system today stem from high prices, not high utilization[52,53]. In its recent assessment of health care spending, the Health Care Cost Institute noted that health care utilization among those with private health insurance has been declining in recent years – instead, growth in spending has been driven by higher prices.

Many had hoped that the introduction of CDHPs, often coupled with tools to make prices more transparent to policyholders, would encourage price shopping. With a very few notable exceptions (switching from brand name to generic drugs[54] and use of lower cost providers for laboratory tests), there is simply no evidence to support this hope. Recent studies indicate that "Members of HDHP and traditional plans are equally likely to price shop for medical care, and they hold similar attitudes about health care prices and quality[55]." The study that found modest evidence of price

---

[50] Fronstin, Paul, Martin J. Sepulveda, and M. Christopher Roebuck. "Medication utilization and adherence in a health savings account-eligible plan." *The American journal of managed care* 19, no. 12 (2013): e400-7.

[51] Brot-Goldberg, Zarek C., Amitabh Chandra, Benjamin R. Handel, and Jonathan T. Kolstad. "What does a deductible do? The impact of cost-sharing on health care prices, quantities, and spending dynamics." *The Quarterly Journal of Economics* 132, no. 3 (2017): 1261-1318.

[52] Health Care Cost Institute. 2016 Health Care Cost and Utilization Report. January 23, 2018. http://www.healthcostinstitute.org/report/.

[53] Papanicolas, Irene, Liana R. Woskie, and Ashish K. Jha. "Health care spending in the United States and other high-income countries." *Jama* 319, no. 10 (2018): 1024-1039.

[54] Fronstin, Paul, and M. Christopher Roebuck. "Brand-Name and Generic Prescription Drug Use After Adoption of a Full- Replacement, Consumer-Directed Health Plan With a Health Savings Account." (2014). https://papers.ssrn.com/sol3/papers.cfm?abstract_id=2414583.

[55] Sinaiko AD, Mehrotra A, Sood N. Cost-Sharing Obligations, High-Deductible Health Plan Growth, and Shopping for Health CareEnrollees With Skin in the Game. *JAMA Intern Med.* 2016;176(3):395–397. doi:10.1001/jamainternmed.2015.7554.

shopping for laboratory tests (suggesting that consumers were aware of and able to navigate the shopping tool) did not detect any evidence of price shopping for office visits.[56] A careful study of the two-year experience of employees of a very large firm that switched to a high deductible plan likewise found no evidence that consumers learned to price shop[57]. The only studies that find robust evidence of price-shopping by beneficiaries are those in which traditional managed care plans use highly-structured pricing arrangements, such as reference pricing, to direct patients to lower cost providers for a very narrow set of conditions. Despite substantial investments in proprietary, commercial, and public transparency tools, there is no evidence that consumers in more loosely structured arrangements such as HDHPs engage in price shopping behavior. Most health care markets are highly concentrated and offer complex products. Most health spending occurs among patients who are very ill and not in a good position to compare costs and quality. The potential for consumers to control prices through shopping is necessarily limited.

Policy Implications

The affordability problems affecting the US health care system today stem from two sources. First, many Americans cannot afford the high deductibles they face in their health insurance plans. Second, the prices of many services within the system are excessively high.

CDHPs offer their greatest value to the highest income taxpayers who face the highest marginal tax rates and have the most discretionary savings available. For these taxpayers, HSAs offer very valuable tax benefits. They also likely reduce the cost of many discretionary services that are not typically covered under health insurance. But high income taxpayers in

[56] Zhang, X., Haviland, A., Mehrotra, A., Huckfeldt, P., Wagner, Z. and Sood, N. (2017), Does Enrollment in High-Deductible Health Plans Encourage Price Shopping?. Health Serv Res. doi:10.1111/1475-6773.12784.

[57] Brot-Goldberg, Zarek C., Amitabh Chandra, Benjamin R. Handel, and Jonathan T. Kolstad. "What does a deductible do? The impact of cost-sharing on health care prices, quantities, and spending dynamics." *The Quarterly Journal of Economics* 132, no. 3 (2017): 1261-1318.

high tax brackets are not the ones facing an affordability problem. For less affluent consumers, CDHPs have not substantially reduced the burden of out-of-pocket costs to date. Given the low level of savings among less affluent Americans, it seems very unlikely that CDHPs will be an affordability solution for this group into the future. Policymakers should look to other solutions to improve financial protections from health care costs for middle income Americans. For example, limiting cost-sharing to levels that are proportional to income, as the Affordable Care Act already does for low income Americans, would be a more effective strategy for addressing the underinsurance problem among middle income Americans.

CDHPs offer even fewer benefits with respect to cost containment and increasing health system efficiency. Well-designed CDHPs can reduce utilization. To date, those reductions in utilization have not focused on the least effective care, but perhaps plans could be further modified to improve access to appropriate services. However, the most important source of high costs in the US health care system today is high prices – not high utilization. High prices, in turn, are to some extent a consequence of increasingly concentrated health care markets, especially for specialized and costly services. While HDHPs reduce utilization, there is no evidence whatsoever that they have been or can be effective in reducing the price of most services. CDHPs will not promote affordability through reducing the overall costs of our healthcare system. Instead, Congress should evaluate new strategies, for example, options that encourage the development of network-based health plans (which can negotiate lower prices through the promise of membership in a network); competitive bidding to enhance price competition in selected sectors; and even increased regulation of prices in highly concentrated markets as alternatives to bring down the prices of health care and enhance affordability for all Americans.

Chairman Roskam. I thank all four of you. I appreciate the perspective. We are the beneficiaries of that, and we will look forward to exploring this further.

I am going to invite Mr. Johnson to inquire.

Mr. Johnson. Thank you, Mr. Chairman.

Mr. Ramthun, welcome. In your testimony, you recommended that Congress allow seniors to continue contributing to HSAs and actually stay off of Medicare for longer.

As a person ages, they generally cost more to care for. So if HSAs are available to seniors, wouldn't you agree that they can help reduce costs to our Medicare system?

Mr. Ramthun. I believe they can absolutely help reduce those costs by staying on a private policy, using their HSA dollars to pay for those expenses, rather than have Medicare pay for those expenses, certainly from the first dollar. So absolutely.

Mr. Johnson. Well, keeping in mind the Medicare Trustees report released yesterday, do you see HSAs as being a part of the solution to save Medicare money?

Mr. Ramthun. I absolutely think HSAs are part of the solution. We need to be looking at all different options, and HSAs are a very good one to include in that list.

Mr. Johnson. Thank you, sir.

I yield back.

Chairman Roskam. Mr. Thompson.

Mr. Thompson. Thank you, Mr. Chairman.

Mr. Eyles, in your written testimony you noted that 82 percent of those plans surveyed offered members healthcare cost information. Can you expand on what you meant by that, what kind of cost information, and how it is used by the consumer?

Mr. Eyles. Sure. Thank you for the question.

So most plans that provide HSAs have tools online that their members can go and use to look at the potential range of costs, for example, of going to a particular healthcare provider or a facility.

It can give a range if you go to one facility versus another, particularly for those that are in network and where an individual is able to benefit from negotiated lower prices, that individuals can find out at least at a general level, and sometimes with great specificity, too, how much a particular healthcare treatment or service might cost depending upon where it is received.

So you can go online, plug in a ZIP Code, plug in a provider, plug in a procedure, and get a range of costs.

Mr. Thompson. And is that somehow juxtaposed with the quality of that procedure?

Mr. Eyles. There is often quality information that is provided at a provider level or a facility level. Obviously, all these tools are different depending upon which plan has developed them. But most of the quality information would allow an individual to compare again, say, the outcome of a hip replacement surgery at one facility versus another.

Mr. Thompson. So the 82 percent, what are you measuring there? Is that 82 percent reflective of quality measurement?

Mr. Eyles. So the 82 percent is around the transparency of cost and price information.

Mr. Thompson. So it is just the cost side. It doesn't necessarily reflect the quality side.

Mr. Eyles. Right. The quality information that we found was about 70 percent had physician-specific quality data and 77 percent had hospital-specific quality data. So it is not a perfect one for one, but overall there is good information to look at both cost, price, and quality.

Mr. Thompson. Okay. Thank you.

Dr. Glied, some of the witnesses have already mentioned that we have watched the volume of HSAs increase dramatically since they were created. But in a 2017 report on employer-sponsored coverage, PricewaterhouseCoopers found that movement to high-deductible health plans loses steam. After shifting healthcare costs to employees for years, the employers are starting to ease off, and that growth in high-deductible employee-based plans is starting to slow.

Can you talk about what might be driving that shift and how much of that should we attribute to the healthcare cost curve versus the economy generally?

Ms. Glied. Thank you for the question.

I think it is difficult to decompose where that change is coming from, but I think one of the factors is growing recognition that it is prices and not utilization that is the main factor that is driving up cost today.

And unfortunately, although many, many plans now include cost and quality information transparency tools, the evidence is very clear that people do not use them and do not find them helpful.

And so if you actually want to do something around prices, just raising people's deductibles doesn't turn out to be the way to do it. And so we see costs continuing to rise in high-deductible plans and insurers and employers looking at other ways to solve these problems.

Mr. Thompson. And then I would ask Mr. Eyles this. When somebody does use the 82 percent, I guess, is the number, those folks, when they do look at the cost, do they get some sort of idea what quality they are getting for that cost?

Ms. Glied. Unfortunately, our metrics of quality that are available to be used on these kinds of tools are just not very good and they are not very credible to most consumers.

So in general, when people's doctor tells them where to go for a checkup or something, they follow their doctor's recommendations and not what it says on the tool. And so there really is a limitation to how these are put into practice.

Mr. Thompson. Thank you. Yield back.

Chairman Roskam. Ms. Jenkins.

Ms. Jenkins. Thank you, Mr. Chairman.

Thank you all for being with us this morning.

Since the inception of flexible spending arrangements and health savings accounts, millions of Americans each year were using these and other similarly tax-preferred health accounts to help reduce their annual healthcare spending.

However, this consumer access changed with the passage of the Affordable Care Act. Consumers are now required to obtain a prescription for over-the-counter medications in order to be eligible for reimbursement under these accounts.

This change, which went into effect January 1 of 2011, severely limits the ability of millions of American families to use funds set aside in their FSAs and HSAs to purchase over-the-counter products, such as those for pain management, smoking cessation, and cold and allergy medications.

Over-the-counter medications are often the frontline treatment for many common illnesses or for maintenance of chronic diseases and should be treated as medically reimbursable healthcare therapies, just as prescription medications are.

A recent study found that over-the-counter medicines save the U.S. healthcare system $102 billion every year through cost savings associated with over-the-counter medicines and avoided visits to the doctor.

Restricting consumers' ability to be reimbursed under FSAs and other tax-preferred accounts imposes an unfair cost increase on individuals and families who are already struggling financially.

So that is why I have introduced legislation, along with Mr. Kind, to restore this benefit, called the Restoring Access to Medication Act. And I am hopeful my colleagues will smile favorably on this legislation soon.

According to an April 2014 study by Nielsen, 75 percent of Americans support changing the law to grant over-the-counter medications tax-preferred preference again.

In fact, the Health Choices Coalition, representing physicians, dentists, consumers, retailers, manufacturers, pharmacies, pharmacists, patients, insurers, and employers large and small, are all in support of restoring this benefit on behalf of millions of Americans.

Americans are being asked to fund more of their healthcare expenses through higher deductibles and copays. So I believe it is more important than ever that cost-effective over-the-counter medicines are treated the same as other eligible medical expenses in tax-preferred healthcare accounts.

I don't know why we should be making it harder for Americans to use their own pretax dollars to purchase these everyday healthcare products.

So with that, Mr. Eyles, shouldn't Congress be making it easier for people to access these safe and effective over-the-counter medications?

Mr. Eyles. We have been supportive of being able to use HSA/FSA funds towards over-the-counter medications. When patients have an option to use something that is over-the-counter, that is a lower cost potentially, not needing to necessarily go and have a physician's office visit, we have been supportive of those kinds of efforts, yes.

Ms. Jenkins. Thank you.

And on that point, so many Kansas communities face the challenges that come with accessing rural healthcare.

So, Mr. Ramthun, do you believe that it makes good public policy sense to require patients, especially rural patients, to seek a doctor's prescription in order to be able to use their tax advantage accounts for medicines that were available over-the-counter?

Mr. Ramthun. Thank you.

I believe it makes no good health policy sense to add cost to the system by seeking an additional office visit just to get something that is available over the counter today.

Ms. Jenkins. Okay. Thank you. I appreciate it.

And with that, Mr. Chairman, I yield back. Chairman Roskam. Mr. Kind.

Mr. Kind. Thank you, Mr. Chairman.

I want to thank the witnesses for coming.

So let me just pick up where my colleague, Ms. Jenkins, just left off. And I am proud to sponsor the Restoring Access to Medicare Act with her. But,

Mr. Eyles, Mr. Ramthun, if you hadn't had a chance to take a look at the specifics of that legislation, I encourage you to do so and give us any feedback in case there is something we might be overlooking.

Mr. Ramthun, let me start with you, because Mr. Johnson already cited the recent Medicare Trustee report that just came out showing that the solvency of Medicare has been reduced by an additional 3 years. In fact, The Washington Post just ran an article in today's paper titled "Key Medicare Fund to Run Out Earlier Than Thought."

Mr. Chairman, I ask unanimous consent to have that inserted in the record at this time.

Chairman Roskam. Without objection, so ordered.

Health & Science

A Crucial Medicare Trust Fund Will Run out Three Years Earlier Than Predicted, New Report Says

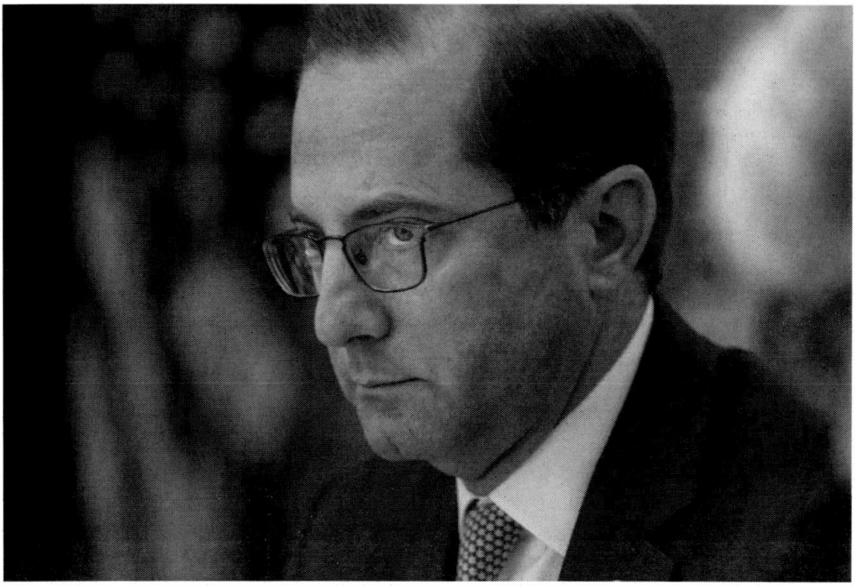

Health and Human Services Secretary Alex Azar is one of the trustees overseeing Medicare. (Melina Mara/The Washington Post)

By Amy Goldstein

June 5

Email the author

The financial future of the part of Medicare that pays older Americans' hospital bills has deteriorated significantly, according to an annual government report that forecasts that the trust fund will be depleted by 2026 — three years sooner than expected a year ago.

The report, issued Tuesday by a quartet of Trump administration officials who are trustees for Medicare and Social Security, reveals that policy changes ushered in by the president and the Republican Congress are weakening the financial underpinnings of the already fragile insurance program.

According to the report, less money will be flowing into the hospital-care trust fund in part because the tax law passed this year will cause the government to collect less in income taxes. In addition, lower wages last year will translate into lower payroll taxes.

As revenue slips, hospital expenses will increase, the report says. A senior government official who briefed reporters on it said that part of that increase is because the tax law will, starting next year, end enforcement of the Affordable Care Act's requirement that most Americans carry health insurance. As a result, hospitals are predicted to have more uninsured patients, in turn requiring the Medicare program to pay more for such uncompensated care.

Unlike in previous years going back decades, none of the trustees — three Cabinet members and the acting Social Security commissioner — attended the report's release at the Treasury Department.

However, Treasury Secretary Steven Mnuchin issued a statement putting a positive spin on the administration's economic agenda, saying that tax cuts, regulatory changes and altered trade policies "will generate the long-term growth needed to help secure these programs and lead them to a more stable path."

Seema Verma, administrator of the Centers for Medicare and Medicaid Services, called on Congress to embrace Medicare proposals in President Trump's budget, saying that they "would strengthen the integrity of the Medicare program." Along with strategies to try to slow spending on prescription drugs, one proposal would shift responsibility for uncompensated care payments from the Medicare program to the Treasury.

The annual reckoning of the stability of the nation's two largest entitlement programs amplifies earlier warnings that both are unsustainable over time. It also urges Congress to revise the programs to ward off the shortfalls soon to "minimize adverse impacts" on the tens of millions of elderly and other vulnerable people who rely on the government help.

The new report's forecast for Social Security is comparatively undramatic. It says that the trust funds that pay benefits to retirees, workers' survivors and people with disabilities can, taken together, be expected to remain solvent until 2034, unchanged from a year ago.

Both programs have long been under pressure because of demographics. The aging of the large baby- boom generation is making up an increasing share of the nation's population, with proportionally fewer working-age Americans chipping in payroll taxes.

Despite officials' contention that Trump's policies would heal the programs' finances, the trustees' report says: "Lawmakers should address these financial challenges as soon as possible." The trustees typically also include two members of the public, but the administration has not filled those positions.

From administration to administration, the trustees' report has for many years been a cautionary note about the financial fragility of the two main programs designed to buffer Americans from poverty in their older years. For more than two decades, presidents of both political parties and Congress have sporadically assembled high-level commissions to explore ways to prolong the solvency of one or both programs. None has led to major changes.

The Trump administration has not placed much focus on the programs' future. The main change since Trump was elected in 2016 has been Congress's action in February to repeal an unpopular aspect of the Affordable Care Act that was intended to have constrained Medicare spending if it rose too high.

The Independent Payment Advisory Board, known as IPAB, was to have been a committee of outside experts with power to slow Medicare's spending if it reached a certain threshold. The board's members were never appointed, and spending levels, as measured by the annual trustees' reports, never reached the critical level.

From before the ACA was passed in 2010, Republican critics erroneously tarred IPAB, which Democrats held out as one of the few teeth in the law to slow health- care expenditures, as a "death panel" that would deny care to the elderly.

In the early years after the ACA was enacted, Obama-era trustees' reports said the law was helping to hold down health-care spending. The report issued Tuesday says that the law had "introduced large policy changes and additional projection uncertainty."

In keeping with efforts by Health and Human Services Secretary Alex Azar — one of the trustees — to usher in new payment methods that reward qualify and cost efficiency, the report says that "if the health sector cannot transition to more efficient models of care delivery and achieve productivity increases, the availability and quality" of care available to older Americans on Medicare will fall.

Sen. Ron Wyden (Ore.), the top Democrat on the Senate Finance Committee, said in a statement, "This chapter should eliminate any doubt that Trump's tax law yanked Medicare closer to insolvency."

House Ways and Means Committee Chairman Kevin Brady (R-Tex.) said in a statement that ensuring the solvency of the two programs "is of the utmost importance. . . . The time is now to come together in a bipartisan manner to address these real challenges."

Mr. Kind. Indicating that with the passage of the recently enacted tax cut, there is going to be a serious drop in revenue that is going to affect the Medicare program, along with the repeal of the individual responsibility aspect of the Affordable Care Act.

The Trustees also cite that there is going to be a huge leap in uninsured and therefore uncompensated care, all of which is going to detrimentally impact the Medicare trust fund by reducing solvency by 3 years to 2026 now.

Mr. Ramthun, you indicated that there might be a role of HSAs to play as far as showing up and bolstering Medicare. What did you have in mind?

Mr. Ramthun. That individuals who are still working at age 65 would be able to take Medicare as a secondary payer.

Today I am self-employed. I must take Medicare as a primary payer. That also applies to workers of small businesses with fewer than 20 employees.

So to give those individuals the option to stay on their employer-based coverage and have Medicare pay their bills on the back end, rather than the front end –

Mr. Kind. You mean past 65 allowing them to stay on their –

Mr. Ramthun. Yes, sir.

Mr. Kind. Okay.

Well, part of the reason you want to get the younger 65s into Medicare is for risk adjustment and spreading the risk, too. So if you will allow more of them just to stay in the private plans, won't that also then jeopardize the long-term solvency and the expense of older and less healthy Medicare patients?

Mr. Ramthun. Medicare does not work like private insurance where you are having to spread risk. Medicare pays claims out of trust fund dollars. So if you have fewer people accessing the trust fund dollars, I would think that would save Medicare money.

Mr. Kind. Ms. Dietel, I think in your testimony you indicated about what the typical HSA participant is contributing every year, from, what $1,000 to $1,500 or so. Is that correct?

Ms. Dietel. Yes, sir.

Mr. Kind. That is substantially below the current contribution limits as they exist today. Is that right?

Ms. Dietel. That is correct.

Mr. Kind. You must have heard Mr. Eyles' testimony earlier, and one of the four points that he said that one of the things we ought to be considering as a committee is perhaps extending the contribution flexibility and therefore raising those contribution limits. What would your response be to that?

Ms. Dietel. I would absolutely support that. I think that participants in HSAs should be able to cover their entire out-of-pocket risk. So there should be parity between the out-of-pocket maximums under the ACA and the contribution limits for health savings accounts.

Mr. Kind. Regardless of income limits right now on an individual, how much they are earning? Does it matter to you?

Ms. Dietel. It doesn't matter to me, although income limits would be one way of addressing alternatives.

Mr. Kind. Ms. Glied, do you have anything to add?

Ms. Glied. I think the concern is that the average of $1,000 includes both people who are funding a lot and putting a lot in their accounts, and those tend to be very high-income people, and people who are putting very little in their accounts.

If we raise that contribution limit, it isn't going to affect the people on the bottom. They are already not bound by the contribution limit. It is just going to allow people at the top to put more money in.

Mr. Kind. Mr. Ramthun, let me ask you, too, one of the groups of people who are getting hammered right now are those in the individual market who don't qualify for any premium tax credits because they are earning too much, and yet the premiums are going up and they are just getting smacked. And you indicated that roughly 10 percent HSA participants are in that individual market.

Is there a way we can, through HSAs, be able to provide some relief to that segment of the 5 percent of the population who is getting hammered in the individual market?

Mr. Ramthun. So some of those individuals already are qualifying for HSA contributions from their employer, so that definitely helps them. By staying in a lower premium plan they can use some of the premium savings to fund their account as well.

Others have suggested using dollars in HSAs to help pay for their premiums, and so that is a provision that is in Congressman Paulsen's bill as well as other bills. So those are ways that HSAs could be used to offset those higher costs.

Mr. Kind. I encourage all of you, as a takeaway today, to keep thinking about how we can better democratize HSAs. I think the problem that many of us have on this side of the dais is that it is weighted to those with more disposable income, those who can afford it, some using it as a tax shelter, because they are generally in good plans and they are generally healthier in regards to the population.

But how do we make this easier for lower to lower-middle-income people to be able to get in and find some tax savings and better manage the cost risks that they face today?

With that, Mr. Chairman, I yield back. Chairman Roskam. Mr. Marchant.

Mr. Marchant. Thank you, Mr. Chairman.

Mr. Ramthun, I come from a congressional district in northeast Texas. We have a very low unemployment rate, well below the national average.

And these workers, who are my constituents, are looking for two things with their hard-earned income: choice in their healthcare decisions and the ability to plan for their future.

This is where HSAs come into play, and I believe that that was the intent of the creation of the HSAs. Would you agree?

Mr. Ramthun. Absolutely, that was the intent.

Mr. Marchant. I have reviewed some of the charts that we have been provided, and it shows that folks in my district are right in what you would call the Goldilocks Zone. They either have HSAs or they are looking at them as a possibility for working that into their health plan and their financial plan.

With insurance premiums rising, we have got to start looking for answers to address out-of-pocket healthcare costs that our constituents face. And one of the most frequent calls that we get from constituent service in our district office is the shockingly high amount of deductible that a normal family faces even in the best plans. And they are looking for every way possible to prepare for an emergency where they have to pay those amounts of money.

Mr. Ramthun or Mr. Eyles, can either of you point to me some specific policy changes that we should be exploring to address this issue and to allow families to use their HSAs in a better way?

Mr. Ramthun. So I will start first. Thank you for the question.

I think the first thing is to allow more of your citizens to take advantage of HSAs. It does give them that flexibility to choose the provider that they want, if it is more cost effective for them to use over-the-counter medicine. So that clearly Ms. Jenkins' bill is an important policy change that needs to go in there.

Helping them get better information about the cost and the quality of those services would give those individuals more information about how they can find better value for their dollars.

So those are two things that I would definitely start with. So, Mr. Eyles.

Mr. Eyles. Thank you for the question, too.

We agree that any policies to make it easier to access HSAs would be positive.

One additional item that I would mention, too, is looking at greater benefit design flexibility to make HSAs an even more attractive option to a broader group of individuals.

Today in America about 60 percent of individuals have a chronic condition of some form or another, and the limitations on how HSA dollars can be used, for example, for certain types of high-value treatments are limited, and you have to go all the way through your deductible.

So policies that would allow individuals to get access to some pre-deductible coverage for high-value services for chronic conditions we also think would be a positive thing.

Mr. Marchant. Ms. Dietel.

Ms. Dietel. Yes, sir. Thank you also for the question.

I think that I would agree strongly with Mr. Eyles' comment that I think some of the waning high-deductible health plan enrollment that you have seen is because employers are needing to be more concerted efforts with regard to chronic care, chronic illness, and value-based design.

And so in some cases they are providing a high-deductible health plan, but it is not HSA qualified because it has some of these other limitations. So certainly expanding access and flexibility for employers in their design of those plans to make them HSA qualified as well would be helpful.

Mr. Marchant. Ms. Glied.

Ms. Glied. I don't think HSAs are going to be the solution to the problems that face the people in your district. I think that what you really want to do is encourage those high-deductible plans to lower their deductibles or to provide exactly the kinds of access to chronic disease services that we would like to see.

I think plugging that through an HSA and expecting somebody to have the savings account on the side in order to pay for their chronic disease prevention is not the way to solve this problem and moving in that direction isn't going to help your constituents.

Mr. Marchant. So you would rather have them have a more expensive plan?

Ms. Glied. The cost of the plan will be a function of what people use. Whether they use it out of their HSA, whether they are using more services or not is the key point here, not whether they are paying for it out of their HSA or not.

Mr. Marchant. I doubt that anyone in my district would agree with that.

Thank you.

Chairman Roskam. Mr. Higgins.

Mr. Higgins. Thank you, Mr. Chairman.

And thank you for being here.

You know, the health savings accounts are helpful in terms of tax treatment, but really does very little to address the underlying problem, which is the rising cost of healthcare and the poor quality.

I have a very simple premise. I think the private insurance companies, their business model is to screw people. They jack up their premiums, they jack up deductibles, they reduce payouts, and they increase premiums.

I think, like anything else in life, particularly with healthcare and in negotiation, it is all about leverage. And I think the Federal Government fails to use the significant leverage that it has under its health insurance programs.

Prescription drugs, the Department of Defense, the Veterans Administration, Medicaid, they negotiate volume discounts, and according to the Commonwealth Fund, they achieve 25 percent savings every year. That is wisely, smartly using the leverage that you have.

Under the Medicare program there are 57 million beneficiaries. From 2010 to 2016 the price per patient, per enrollee cost increased about 1.3 percent as compared during the same period for private insurance 3.5 percent.

So I think the Federal Government needs to do a much better job using its leverage to drive down the cost of healthcare and drive up the quality.

I am particularly concerned about the population between the ages of 50 and 64. They get hammered in terms of health insurance premiums on the exchanges. They are to this century what the traditional Medicare population was to the 20th century, and that is that insurance companies have every opportunity to provide good insurance products for that segment of the population and didn't want to because it wasn't profitable for them to provide insurance that was affordable and good for people that are older and statistically sicker.

So now it is 50 to 64 that gets hammered. We have an obligation to try to help them.

So, Dr. Glied, I would ask you, I have a bill that would simply allow those between the ages of 50 and 64-1/2 to buy in at their own cost into the Medicare program, which is the insurance. Medicare is fully compliant with the essential benefits of the Affordable Care Act.

Why, as a healthcare economist, why in God's name wouldn't the Federal Government use its leverage to provide, first of all, relief to this segment of the population, of which there are 60 million people? If you divide that by the number of congressional districts, that comes up to 138,000 people per district – and that segment of the population votes.

So why aren't we using that leverage to provide at the very least relief to a population, 50 to 64-1/2, that is getting clobbered?

Ms. Glied. Thank you. Thank you for the question.

I commend you for paying attention to this population. I think it is a population that really needs the Federal Government to be thinking through what are the best ways to address it, and public options might be one of the things that should be on the table for that population.

I think we need to work through the benefits and the costs of a variety of different strategies to address that group, making sure that we maintain the viability of the Medicare program and trying to really figure out what is going to work best, both for that population and I think also for people with lower incomes that are at ages below that.

But I think really thinking about the Federal Government's power to establish prices and to affect prices in the marketplace, not only the exchange marketplaces but in the healthcare system throughout, I think is really an important direction for policy to take.

Mr. Higgins. And, Doctor, I would say this, that the second beneficial effect to allowing people to buy into the Medicare program, it would allow private insurance companies to compete for that more desirable, because of less utilization, that 27 to 50 population, which you would have better products that would promote things like healthy lifestyles and prevention, thus creating a healthier future Medicare population.

I mean, look, this is not ideological; it is arithmetical. And I think we have to take a commonsense approach when it comes to healthcare because the center will not hold. We cannot sustain 7 to 8 percent annual growth over the next 10 years.

Thanks very much. Yield back. Chairman Roskam. Mrs. Black.

Mrs. Black. Thank you, Mr. Chairman. And I want to thank you for bringing the panel here today to talk about something that we don't talk about often enough, and that is some ideas outside of what the traditional ideas are.

So for 8 years now, everywhere I go in my district, people will tell me stories about how ObamaCare's heavy hand has cost them money and has hurt their healthcare.

And in Tennessee, we see the collapse of ObamaCare is really having some dire circumstances for our citizens. We see massive premium increases that are making health insurance unaffordable for more and more Tennesseeans. And we also see that the rising deductibles are really hurting them and making it even harder for them to get the services when they do pay the high premiums.

I think that we can't continue to do nothing. We have got to look outside of the box and look to some things that maybe haven't been quite as public as some of the other products that are out there.

So we have to continue to work to empower individual families and allow them to make those decisions for themselves based on what best fits their needs, what best fits their wants, and what also best fits their pocketbook or their budget.

Now, as a nurse for more than 45 years, I know that a central challenge of reforming the healthcare system is finding policy solutions to lower the cost of healthcare, while also increasing access to healthcare. I think that is part of what this discussion is about today, and I thank you for being here.

So while we work toward a permanent solution to bring relief to the American people, these healthcare savings accounts do empower individuals to be able to invest and use their healthcare dollars however they best see fit.

By expanding these HSAs to cover certain low-cost, high-value services like chronic care services below the deductible, not only can we help those with chronic conditions better manage their care, but we can also save the healthcare system billions of dollars through better medication adherence.

The Chronic Disease Management Act of 2018 that I have sponsored with my colleague on the other side of the aisle, Mr. Blumenauer, is a simple bipartisan measure that we introduced.

Mr. Eyles, I want to start with you. You mentioned in your testimony that covering high-value services can help reduce long-term costs. Can you expand on some of the benefits of allowing that first dollar of coverage for chronic care, both for patients and for the healthcare system overall?

Mr. Eyles. Sure. Thank you for the question, Congresswoman. And we support your legislation. We think it is an important step to improve HSAs to make chronic conditions eligible for pre-deductible services.

And as I mentioned, with 60 percent of Americans having at least one chronic condition, over 40 percent have two or more, ways that we can provide some more flexibility to provide access to high-value services, I think one of the best examples, whether it be in the area of diabetes or cardiovascular disease conditions, to be able to provide treatments pre-deductible can have the effect of keeping people healthier longer, preventing them from using much more expensive specialty services, hopefully keep them out of the hospital.

Better management, for example, of blood glucose levels over time could definitely lead to better outcomes for patients with diabetes and making the healthcare system more efficient and keeping them out of higher-cost areas.

So we are very supportive of trying to provide access to those types of services that are proven to work, that have strong evidence, that we know really do have an impact on the lives of patients and the overall healthcare system and costs.

Mrs. Black. Well, I thank you for that.

I can tell you, as a visiting nurse, that when I would go see my patients and they had diabetes, I would take their blood sugar and we would see that it would be elevated, and I would say, "Are you using your medication?"

They would say, "Well, I am just using half of it because I don't have a whole lot of it left. So I am saving some for tomorrow or the next day."

I would say, "It doesn't exactly work that way."

But I appreciate your comments and appreciate the fact that you do support our measure.

Thank you. And I yield back. Chairman Roskam. Ms. Chu.

Ms. Chu. Dr. Glied, I would like to ask you about the HSAs as it pertains to women.

In your written testimony, you mentioned that one concern with the high-deductible health plans and HSAs is that, in practice, these plans haven't reduced the burden of out-of-pocket costs for consumers. Although the lower premiums can make insurance seem more affordable, these plans rely on consumers' ability to plan for medical emergencies, which often can't be predicted.

So then, let's talk about women and pregnancy and their out-of-pocket costs. Because 9-months pregnancies often span 2 plan years, women would have to hit their plan's deductibles twice within the course of a single pregnancy. And if a women has one these plans when she gives birth, she could, depending on the complications, face over $20,000 in out-of-pocket costs under high-deductible health plans.

Even if a family has dutifully been saving for the arrival of a new child, medical complications can put the child's birth well outside the scope of the family's savings.

Another unforeseen cost that often shocks new mothers occurs when the mother receives care from an anesthesiologist who is out of the plan's network during delivery.

The mother, of course, most often has no control over which anesthesiologist is available to care for her. It is unreasonable to assume that she would be shopping for an anesthesiologist while she is in the delivery room giving birth. And even if the hospital and OB/GYN are in network, the anesthesiologist might not be.

While being served by an out-of-network doctor is a pervasive issue amongst many types of plans, it is particularly impactful to those who have high-deductible plans because they are charged with higher out-of-pocket costs than those with other health plans.

So can you discuss how these high-deductible health plans shifts the costs to a consumer, especially in the case of an unexpected medical cost, like a complicated pregnancy?

Ms. Glied. Thank you very much.

I think that is exactly the problem with high-deductible health plans, which is that, even if we exempt various services at the bottom end, people who actually have something wrong with them or really need costly services, like pregnant women, are going to be the ones who wind up paying a lot of money out of pocket.

And very, very few people have enough money in their health savings accounts, and virtually no middle-income people have enough money in their health savings accounts, to pay those deductibles for an expense like pregnancy. That is just not a realistic expectation.

The second point you made, about seeing an out-of-network anesthesiologist, points to the big problem with thinking about using transparency tools and quality tools of the type that we are offering to get people to shop.

There is a real limit to how much shopping we can plausibly expect happens in the healthcare system. When you are lying on that table, you are not checking your phone to see which anesthesiologist is in network. And that is just not a good way to build a healthcare system.

Ms. Chu. In fact, given the fact that half of all births in the U.S. are unplanned, it seems to me that these consumer-directed health plans would leave a number of families behind when it comes to the birth of a child.

So, Dr. Glied, would you say that these types of health plans are adequate substitutes for comprehensive health coverage?

Ms. Glied. Absolutely not. And there is no evidence at all that providing an HSA on top of a high-deductible health plan undoes that difference. In fact, that is the whole point of a high-deductible health plan.

Ms. Chu. And let me ask about prescription drugs, because right now $1 out of every $6 spent on healthcare in this country is spent on prescription drugs. But a recent study by the Pharmacy Benefit Consultants found that over the past 14 months 20 prescription drugs have been seeing price increases of over 200 percent.

So do these plans do anything to address the skyrocketing underlying price of these drugs?

Ms. Glied. I don't think there is any evidence to suggest that they do any more than any other plans do to reduce the price of those drugs. The only thing that they really do is shift more of that cost onto the patients who need the drugs.

Ms. Chu. Thank you. I yield back.

Chairman Roskam. Mr. Paulsen.

Mr. Paulsen. Thank you, Mr. Chairman, and for holding the hearing. There actually has been some really instructive testimonies today.

Look, I mean we already know that healthcare savings accounts are becoming more and more popular. At least 22 million Americans are using these HSAs. A lot of Minnesotans are actually using healthcare savings accounts. The average income level of the folks that are using them is less than $60,000. These are middle-income folks, average middle class Americans that are actually interested in making sure they are using their own healthcare dollars for their own healthcare needs.

You talked a little bit about some of the incentives that are needed. Some of us have legislation that actually have more incentives to use HSAs, and that gives some more flexibility to patients, removing limitations for those who may have chronic conditions.

I want to ask one other question regarding this concept of direct primary care that has become more and more popular that I am hearing from primary physicians, family physicians, and actually now a lot of employers whose employees are using this model, where they do a monthly or a quarterly subscription with a primary physician.

They have that doctor-patient relationship where they can see them as often as they want and really have that close connectivity, which has been lost, unfortunately, in a lot of reforms in healthcare recently.

So Representative Blumenauer and I have introduced bipartisan legislation together, which allows an HSA to reimburse or to cover that expense for direct primary care.

Mr. Ramthun, I am wondering if you can just talk a little bit about what is it that makes these direct primary care arrangements more and more popular among individuals and employers and unions, for that matter? And why should HSAs be a component of that? Can you elaborate on that?

Mr. Ramthun. Thank you, Congressman Paulsen.

I think people are looking for, for lack of a better term, a medical home, a relationship with a physician which seems to be increasingly challenged these days.

Many physicians are retiring. We have seen many urgent and retail clinics pop up in their place where it is convenient to get healthcare. It may even be more cost effective. But our primary care physician has retired and we are looking for somebody else.

So I think we need to recognize that these relationships are changing between patients and their physicians, and not everybody pays on a fee-for-service basis anymore.

So HSAs are not currently flexible enough to allow those types of relationships to be paid from an HSA. And in fact we believe that the coverage, if you will, that relationship between the doctor and the patient, actually cancels their HSA eligibility even when they are enrolled in the right type of health insurance plan.

So your bill addresses that and would go a long way to helping those people out.

Mr. Paulsen. Mr. Eyles, maybe you can explain this. Would some of your members see this as a similar flexible arrangement that would serve a need in the population similar to chronic care?

Mr. Eyles. I think many of our members have been very focused on ways to enhance access to primary care.

I think the benefits of having a relationship with a primary care provider are very well known. And trying to make sure that that relationship is close so that there can be care coordination, so that there can be ongoing treatment I think is a very positive step.

We want to make sure that that relationship, that there aren't barriers to having good relationships with primary care physicians. And so things that support primary care relationships to make sure that people get access to lower-cost care, to get continuity of care, are generally viewed as positive things.

Mr. Paulsen. Yeah, thank you.

And, Mr. Ramthun, you can offer a quick comment. But I think as we have had this discussion here, as we have had over the years, of course, there are a lot of reasons why healthcare costs are high and they have been a challenge for families and individuals and small businesses.

But one of the biggest contributing factors is that consumers tend to be disconnected from their healthcare spending. There is usually an insurer that is acting as that middle person between the patient and often the cost of the service, and figuring how much something actually costs can be a challenge in healthcare.

Would you agree or disagree that HSAs are actually a good tool to help reduce costs in our current system right now?

Mr. Ramthun. I believe they are a good tool, even though others may disagree.

I certainly pay a lot more attention to what things cost. Sometimes I don't know that in advance and I find out after the fact and I have wished I had known and was able to ask other questions like, do I even need that? Because I might have decided differently.

I do think that we have a long way to go in our healthcare system as to making consumers aware of those differences, the quality that sometimes is inversely related to the cost of the care. So we are making headway.

But everybody has these challenges. It is not something that is unique to HSA qualified plans. Those individuals are most financially impacted by doing so, though.

Mr. Paulsen. Mr. Chairman, I think that in having this hearing today, there is a recognition that there is not some silver bullet magic answer to solve all these challenges, but this is clearly a piece of the puzzle that can make a big difference for consumers.

And I yield back.

Chairman Roskam. Thank you.

Mr. Kelly.

Mr. Kelly. Thank you, Mr. Chairman.

Thank you all for being here.

First of all, I just want to approach this from a little different place because I actually own a business. I am an automobile dealer, and we do buy health insurance for the people that we work with: our associates.

So I think sometimes you can debate this stuff, you can keep talking about it, but unless you are actually on the field doing it, it is a little bit different, because people have these ideas. I read a study that says this doesn't work.

So I do know that for people who own their own businesses and want to take care of the people they work with every day, the way we have to go is to come up with mutual success.

Mr. Blumenauer, I didn't realize you are on all these bills. You are a champion. I knew that already.

But Earl and I have a bill called the Bipartisan HSA Improvement Act that reduces barriers, expands access, and makes healthcare more affordable. This commonsense bill has already been endorsed by 60 organizations.

I want to go with it not from the notes that I have here, because I have been listening to everybody and I get it. But I want some of you to weigh in on something right now.

It is my belief, and some of you are in my age group, but there used to be an advertisement on TV for Fram oil filters. Do you remember the guy holding the filter? And he would say, "You can pay me now or you can pay me later." He meant, if you change the oil in your car or your truck and you change the filter, that truck or car is going to run a lot better and a lot more economical.

I think it is the same thing with people. I wonder all the time as we look at what is happening as a society, preventative maintenance is probably the cure or one of the cures to making sure we have more healthy communities and a population.

So I look at this, and I just am trying to figure it out, if you can all weigh in on this. I think HSAs are the way to go. I think that when you allow people to do what they want to do with their own money and make it available to them to do something ahead of them time with pre-tax money, they are going to make decisions that make sense for them.

And people who say they don't really look at it that way, I would just say that you have got to come home with me and look at the 56 people that work at our dealership right now. They make really smart decisions, especially when it is their money.

So I think the HSAs, while not the cure-all, and I know it is not, but we also have a piece for the healthcare sharing ministries, where faith-based people who really believe that helping each other kind of goes back to the basics of who we are.

But if you can each weigh in a little bit on this idea that if we are going to look at this, because a lot of people right now, I have got to tell you, we have paid almost $600,000 this year for our insurance for 56 of the 127 people that we work with every day.

Now, they have an insurance card, but they have very little coverage, and that is because in order to keep it at 600,000 grand, we had to do things with deductibles and copays.

Now, we are trying to come up with a way to help them. How do we help them with their copays? How do we help them with their deductibles? How do we do that? HSAs are a way to do that with those pre-tax dollars.

But I want to get to wellness programs and, in addition, exercise. We need to start looking at nutrition, too, because part of wellness is eating right to begin with. So each of you can weigh in.

How could that fit in with the HSAs, and allowing people to make commonsense decisions for their own health every day and for their families, which I believe mothers and fathers do. Just give us a little bit of a flavor of that, because I know it is not the cure-all for everything, but it has got to be incredibly important. This preventative maintenance is incredibly important.

Mr. Ramthun. Well, I will start. Thank you for the question.

I believe employers are starting to recognize that, that we need to look at employees' health more holistically. And so some of them are using incentive-based programs – some are tied to HSAs, some are not – to encourage their employees to lead healthier lifestyles so that these costs are reduced down the long-term.

I think Ms. Dietel and Mr. Eyles can talk about some of these specific programs that they are aware of where employers have done just that.

Mr. Kelly. Okay.

Mr. Eyles. So thank you for the question. And we, too, have supported your legislation. We signed on to a letter that recommends that this bill be enacted because it is a very positive step.

We agree that providing more access to preventive care and treatment and services, whether it be through innovative wellness programs, through telemedicine, and being able to provide access to lower-cost care that is more convenient, to your point, that gets to the right care at the right time, especially when it is done earlier, can offset the need for much more expensive treatments and services down the road. And we are very supportive of those efforts.

Ms. Dietel. Yes, Congressman. Thank you for the question.

It is important to recognize that the Affordable Care Act for both high-deductible health plans and other coverage requires first-dollar preventive services. So I think that the issue is really for better communication to participants that they have access to these services already. I think that is one critical component, at least in working with our clients, that we help them communicate more effectively their plans.

But I think also, to my colleagues' points here, employers are trying all sorts of innovative things. As we have discussed, value-based design. They want to help people with chronic conditions be healthier. They want to provide wellness incentives.

And, again, I think this is communicating. And sometimes, unfortunately, the people who are going to commit to wellness efforts are people that already go to the gym and already eat right and those kinds of things.

Mr. Kelly. Right, right. So we have got to get more people on board.

Ms. Dietel. It is helping those that need those chronic illnesses move –

Mr. Kelly. Just one more thing. I know my time is up. But honestly, we always talk about the cost of doing this and how it is going to affect our tax revenue. I would like somebody to do a study on the cost of not doing it and what we are doing to our total population.

Long-range, you can pay me now or pay me later, I think we are reaching a point right now where there is no such thing. The dollar amount is so crazy, that if we don't get people healthier earlier on, we have great problems.

So thank you all for being here.

Mr. Chairman, thank you for allowing me to go over. And Earl, thanks for being on everything.

Chairman Roskam. Mr. Blumenauer.

Mr. Blumenauer. Thank you, Mr. Kelly.

Well, I do think that we have mechanisms now with health savings accounts that have been embraced by a variety of people for a variety of reasons.

I appreciate some of the cautionary notes about how are we getting the maximum impact for healthcare with them. And I think those are valid. And I think we ought not to just rush in to wildly increased limits and not look at the consequences.

I think program design is very, very important. And I think there is common ground here. We can do things. And Mrs. Black and I have been harassing people about this for a number of years, and with good research out of Michigan, that that makes sense.

One other item that I have been working with Mr. Paulsen on deals with the arbitrary definition of direct primary care that it somehow is a whole new health plan, and some people have taken advantage. Dismissively, it is called concierge service.

But I have had interesting experience with a physician who simply doesn't take insurance, but he is able to provide very intense personal attention because he is not dealing with all the overhead and whatnot. It is not for everybody, but it has an important role. But it was interesting to me to find out that that doesn't qualify for participation in a program.

Beyond that I was – I can take that, life goes on – but to find out that they couldn't undertake the direct primary care for employers who for a nominal sum, $50, $100 a year, something like that, be able to provide that personal connection, and that it would be deemed somehow it was a different healthcare program, and they were denied.

And so I think this would have nominal impact on the overall cost, but it would have significant impact in terms of being able to use an innovative approach that I have no doubt in my mind would reduce overall healthcare expenses and improve outcomes for patients and doctors who are on the assembly line.

Every 11 minutes there is a new patient coming in, and there is so much churn, inefficiency, it is not the best care, it is hard on patients, but it complies with rules of the road.

So I would respectfully suggest that we ought to move forward with a package of some of these things that are not controversial, that don't depend on whether or not we are going to have the Affordable Care Act, we don't have to blow up ObamaCare to be able to move forward with these, and we don't have to open the floodgates to more and more benefits for people who may not need it.

But more to the point, it wouldn't be the most efficient way of allocating scarce dollars, because someday we are going to get back to thinking about allocating scarce dollars, after we have spent trillions of dollars here at this dais in a matter of minutes. This is something that can bring us together.

I would just for the record, Mr. Chairman, I would like to submit a statement for one other thing that speaks to Mr. Kelly's big picture item. And we have had a lot of fun talking about things like that.

One of the big picture items that concerns me is that we have had 293 hearings since your team has been in charge. We have had 5 minutes devoted to infrastructure finance. And this has serious health implications for our Nation, having infrastructure that is falling apart as we fall behind.

It is not just traffic safety, it is water quality. There are any number of areas. Air pollution.

And if we actually maybe spent a week or 2 listening to certified small people, starting with the U.S. Chamber of Commerce and the AFL-CIO and the Truckers Association, head of the Automobile Dealers Association, engineers, local government, we could talk about what would happen if our committee met our responsibility dealing with infrastructure finance which would have dramatic healthcare consequences, not just creating millions of family-wage jobs, but actually improving air quality, water quality, traffic safety. It would make a difference for healthcare in this country.

So I would just like to submit a statement to the record. Chairman Roskam. Without objection, so ordered.

Mr. Blumenauer. I like this hearing. I enjoy what we are talking about. Hope we can move forward. But I hope we can find more than 5 minutes to talk about a threat to our Nation's health with the decline of infrastructure.

Thank you. I appreciate it.

Chairman Roskam. Good segue way.

Ms. Sewell.

Ms. Sewell. Thank you, Mr. Chairman.

And I want to thank our witnesses today.

I have a doctor in my State, Dr. John Waits, who runs the only rural family medicine residency in my State. He grew up in a conservative household and interned at a think tank in 1993 where he fought Democratic healthcare reform efforts.

He studied medicine, thinking he would serve as a missionary abroad, but instead he found himself at a hospital in a rural part of Alabama, Centreville, and he runs the only family medicine practice there.

He told my office before that he realized quickly that he had a lot of patients who were underemployed, without a vehicle, chronically ill, or food insecure, and that these Americans would reap benefits if they had the money to put in these tax-free savings accounts. But that money was nonexistent for lots and lots of these patients.

He often says that he remembers realizing 2 weeks into his post-residency that he hadn't met a single patient for whom a health savings account would solve anything.

Mr. Chairman, I ask for unanimous consent to submit this article in the record about my district and Dr. Waits. It is called "The Health Care System is Leaving the Southern Black Belt Behind."

Chairman Roskam. Without objection, so ordered.

THE HEALTH CARE SYSTEM IS LEAVING THE SOUTHERN BLACK BELT BEHIND

https://fivethirtyeight.com/features/the-health-care-system-is-leaving-the-southern-black-belt-behind

Sitting outside of a Starbucks on the corner of a strip mall in Tuscaloosa late last year, Dr. Remona Peterson described her hometown of Thomaston, Alabama, population 400. "Everybody loves our grocery store. That's, like, our pride," she said with a laugh. She was in Tuscaloosa, Alabama's fifth-largest city, finishing her medical residency when Dave's Market opened in an old Thomaston high school gym last year. Peterson said it became the only place to buy groceries for miles in any direction, and it was one of the few changes to the town she can remember from the last three decades.

Peterson wants to be a part of positive change in the region, which is why she's back after a circuitous journey through medical school. She was valedictorian of her 29-person high school class and graduated summa cum laude from Tuskegee University, where she earned a full scholars hip and the university's distinguished scholars award. She went on to medical school and got the residency in Tuscaloosa. It was her first choice; she felt that the University of Alabama would best prepare her for her long-term goal: to add her name to the short list of African-American doctors working in the Alabama Black Belt who were also born and raised there.

The Black Belt refers to a stretch of land in the U.S. South whose fertile soil drew white colonists and plantationowners centuries ago. After hundreds of thousands of people were forced there as slaves, the region became the center of rural, black America. Today, the name describes predominantly rural counties where a large share of the population is African-American. The area is one of the most persistently poor in the country, and residents have some of the most limited economic prospects. Life expectancies are among the shortest in the U.S., and poor health outcomes are common. This article is part of a series examining these disparities.

The disparities partly stem from a lack of access to care - but access is a complicated notion. Early in the Republican efforts to repeal and replace the Affordable Care Act, the GOP homed in on the idea, saying the party wanted to guarantee "access to health care" for everyone. But the ongoing national policy conversation has hinged on insurance coverage, the main issue tackled by both the Affordable Care Act and the current GOP efforts. Yes, measuring who's insured illuminates one way by which people have access to the health care system, but it's only part of the picture. The term "access to health care" has a standardized federal definition that's much broader: "the timely use of personal health services to achieve the best health outcomes." And there's a list of metrics to measure it. Researchers consider structural barriers, such as distance to a hospital or how many health professionals work in an area, to be important. As are metrics that gauge whether a patient can find a health care provider that she trusts and can communicate with well enough to get the services she needs.

Southern states have health outcomes that are among the worst in the U.S. overall, and they have some of the largest in-state health disparities, according to County Health Rankings, an annual report from the Robert Wood Johnson Foundation and the University of Wisconsin. Transportation options are limited, and health care worker shortages are routine. In Alabama, Black Belt counties have fewer primary care physicians, dentists and mental health providers per resident than other counties. They also tend to have the highest rates of uninsured people.

Poverty rates, which are associated with limited access to care, are also high.

Becoming a Doctor in the Black Belt

Peterson knows these challenges well, but she objects to people viewing the region as hopeless. "The Black Belt is just so much in need. I don't want to be looked at ... as though people are dumb. And people do look at us like that," Peterson told me. "Some people just need opportunity. Like me, I needed that opportunity. Someone just gotta give us a chance."

Peterson likes to acknowledge the help she got during her quest to become a doctor. Her impressive resume masks the deeply rooted challenges she encountered growing up. Her parents were teachers, which gave her family financial stability, but the largely segregated public schools she attended had little in the way of supplies or technology. She had some great teachers, including a chemistry teacher who Peterson credits with her love of science, but she was shocked by what her classmates already knew when she reached college. 'Tm looking around the room like, 'how do people know this?' I was lost," she said. She went on to win an award from the university in her freshman year, for best chemistry and math student. Though she was always a straight- A student, testing wasn't her forte, and she had trouble with the MCAT, the exam required for entry to most medical schools.

She enrolled in a master's program in rural and community health, trying to buy time to lift her test scores. She finished the master's, but didn't raise her test scores, so she ended up at medical school on a Caribbean island, working simultaneously on an MBA that allowed her to receive some U.S. student loans to pay tuition. After two years she was back in the U.S., her family tapped out of money, trying to figure out how to pay for the rest of her degree.

Then, Peterson was connected to a hospital near her hometown via a farming cooperative she'd worked with while getting her master's. She explained her situation to the hospital administrator, and, thrilled by the idea of a doctor from the area coming back to work in the community, he struck an unusual deal: Greene County Health System, about midway between her hometown and Tuscaloosa, would pay for the rest of Peterson's education if she agreed to work there after she graduated. She readily accepted. She found a program she could finish from within the U.S., and in 2014, she graduated from medical school.

Insurance and Access

Greene County Hospital is in a low-slung brick building a couple of blocks from the center of Eutaw, Alabama. The town has hollowed out over the years, though its past riches are still on display in the Kirkwood plantation house, and empty stores line the main square. The hospital was hit hard by the county's shrinking population, which is about 8,400-less than a third of what it was in 1860, when more than three-quarters of the population were slaves. Jobs and potential patients have evaporated. But the dwindling population isn't all that makes it hard for the hospital to stay afloat, CEO Elmore Patterson III said.

Greene County is high on poverty and low on resources; centuries' worth of inequalities have led to major health disparities. And the hospital suffers from problems plaguing rural health systems across the country - too many uninsured people, patients who are sick and have few resources, and aging infrastructure.

The mix of people who use the hospital's services also poses a financial challenge. People with money and private insurance mostly travel to larger cities to seek care, which means most people using Greene County Health System are uninsured or on public insurance like Medicaid or Medicare. About 7 percent of patients have commercial insurance, Patterson said, and about 8 percent have no insurance at all. This affects the hospital's bottom line.

Doctors, policy experts and even some state officials say an important but controversial first step would improve access to health care: expanding Medicaid.

Nearly half of the people who use the Greene County Health System now are on Medicaid, the public health insurance program for low-income people. Having so many patients on Medicaid is a stress on the system because the program offers lower reimbursement rates for care than other health insurance providers, Patterson said. But from the hospital's perspective, it's far better than a patient having no insurance at all.

Alabama allows broad access to Medicaid for children; anyone under age 18 in a family earning below S12 percent of the federal poverty level, or about $76,000 for a family of four, qualifies.

Technically the 312 percent threshold is the income cut off for the Children's Health Insurance Program, or CHIP. Children up to 18 qualify for Medicaid if they are in a family earning 141 percent of the federal poverty level. The two programs are combined in statistics cited throughout this story.

But Alabama is one of the most conservative states when it comes to access for adults. Healthy, childless adults aren't eligible for Medicaid, no matter their income, and parents must make below 13 percent of the federal poverty line to qualify. "You don't have any healthy people on Medicaid in the state of Alabama," Patter son said. That means a lot of care and little money to pay for it, he said.

Even though Medicaid doesn't pay a lot, the uninsured patients are even more of a strain on the system. Adult men working for low hourly wages without benefits have no realistic way to buy health insurance, and they often end up in the emergency department when something goes wrong, Patterson said. That was meant to change with the Affordable Care Act. The law was written to expand Medicaid in every state, in theory reducing the number of uninsured people using hospital services, and so it cut some of the federal government's reimbursements for care provided to the uninsured. But after the Supreme Court ruled that states could choose whet her to expand Medicaid, Alabama, like most of the Black Belt states.

Arkansas and Louisiana have expanded, while Texas, Mississippi, Alabama, Georgia, North Carolina, South Carolina, Florida and Virginia have not.

Said no thanks. The result has been less support from the federal government for uninsured patients, many of whom would qualify for Medicaid under the expansion.

"The Black Belt is a road map," said Patrick Sullivan, a professor at the Rollins School of Public Health at Emory University who previously worked on HIV surveillance at the Centers for Disease Control and Prevention. "That's what's so tragic and so compelling. It's an endgame depiction of what happens when you have social and structural inequalities. It's the vestiges of slavery and inequality, and in the long run those things do play out as health inequalities." Sullivan and colleagues have studied why HIV rates are so much higher among African-Americans and Latinos than other racial groups.

The reasons for the high HIV rates in the Deep South are complex and are discussed in detail in a recent story in The New York Times Magazine.

And found that health insurance is the most important mediating factor. People in both racial/ ethnic groups are more likely to be poor and have less education, which are related barriers, but insurance coverage is where the local and federal government could improve access to treatment, Sullivan said.

Since most Southern states chose not to expand Medicaid, there's no clear way to dismantle that barrier. And a GOP push not only to roll back the expansion but also to shift costs onto states for the longstanding parts of the program could leave even more people uninsured or with access to fewer services.

Structural Barriers and Access

Greene County Hospital has *been* struggling for years. Its operating profit margin is - 19.5 percent, according to an evaluation by the Chartis Center for Rural Health, making it one of the worst-performing rural hospitals.

The Chart is estimate is for the hospital. Greene Count y Health System as a whole has about a -13 percent operating profit margin, Patterson said.

Financially speaking, in Alabama. Care is often more expensive to provide in rural settings, where hospitals are too small to negotiate the best prices for supplies and equipment. The bills the GOP has proposed to replace the ACA would make the problem worse: Cuts to Medicaid would disproportionately hit rural hospitals, which largely depend on funding from the program.

Other rural hospitals are collapsing under the weight of these problems, too. Nearly 80 have permanently closed in the U.S. since 2010, according to data compiled by the Sheps Center for Health Services Research at the University of North Carolina. Alabama alone has lost five of *54* rural hospitals since 2010; several more, like Greene County's, operate in the red.

Having to travel long distances for essential care can be a barrier to access. People who live far from emergency rooms are more likely to die from emergencies such as heart disease or accidents. People in rural areas also frequently live farther from pharmacies and are less likely to receive preventive services. For example, there is no prenatal care available in Greene County, Patterson said, which is a problem in much of the Black Belt and in other rural counties across the U.S. The Greene County Health System can provide a few basics, such as prenatal vitamins, but pregnant women must travel for an ultrasound. That's also the case when it's time for women to have their babies. It's nearly an hour-and-a-half drive to Tuscaloosa from Peterson's hometown, Thomaston, but the nearby labor and delivery unit in Demopolis closed in 2014. During Peterson's residency, she met women who had given birth in the car while making the drive to a hospital.

States are looking for solutions, alternatives to full-service rural hospitals, to create new kinds of geographical access to care. Some places are considering the use of freestanding emergency departments. There's also a movement toward allowing nurse practitioners to take charge of more services than they are currently allowed to provide. But these ideas require additional research and regulatory changes. In the meantime, rural hospital systems are often the only option for communities when an emergency strikes. Patients need facilities, and those facilities need to be reimbursed for care if they are going to survive.

Some places have found creative ways to buck the closure trend. In Centreville, just north of the state-defined Black Belt, the Cahaba Medical Care facility serves a largely low-income population, and a quarter of patients are black. It's attached to a count y hospital, and together they opened a labor and delivery unit in 2015. It was the rebirth of a facility that had closed about *15* years before. The man who led that effort, Dr. John Waits, also runs the only rural family medicine residency in Alabama and is part of a small but tenacious group of Alabamians trying to expand training options for doctors who want to work in rural communities.

Waits, who is white, grew up in a conservative, Christian Alabama family with a father who was a surgeon. His conservative beliefs extended to the health care system, and he spent a summer as an intern at the Family Research Council, fighting Hillary Clinton's 1993 effort to overhaul health insurance. He then studied medicine, assuming he'd work as a missionary abroad. But after his residency, he found himself at a hospital in Centreville, a rural town southeast of Tuscaloosa. He remembers being blown away by the disconnect between conservative policy proposals and the conditions in the community. "I distinctly remember two weeks post-residency, sitting down on the sofa and thinking, 'I haven't met a single patient for whom a health savings account will solve anything,'" he said, referencing a cornerstone of conservative health policy that allows people to put money aside tax-free to pay for medical services . He says it quickly became apparent to him that the state needed to get insurance to the poorest Alabamians and that sometimes the coverage would need to be free.

Waits and several partners set about opening a new clinic, one that would provide a full range of health services to an underserved community and would charge on a sliding scale based on patient income.

The clinic is a Federally Qualified Health Center, which means it qualifies for higher reimbursements from the federal government but must meet certain criteria, including this sliding scale for fees.

Today, the staff of Cahaba provides mental health, primary, and pediatric care. Its staff also see patient s at the county hospital's nursing facility, labor and delivery, and inpatient units.

The clinic won Waits accolades around the state, including from the governor's mansion. It also helped land him a spot on a task force that former Gov. Robert Bentley convened to find ways to improve access to health care in the state, with a focus on rural communities. "We've got unanimous resolution that it's Medicaid," Waits told me late last fall, before Bentley resigned because of a sex scandal. In a carefully worded report, the group suggested that the state "must move forward at the earliest opportunity to close Alabama's health coverage gap."

"Nothing happens without Medicaid," Waits said. "It is the No. l, the No. 2, it is the top 10 solutions."

Years of work have also taught Waits that a functional system has to at least be able to provide preventive care for women and children. "It's a whole nother thing trying to get the men in for their colonoscopies. But if the kids are getting in for their vaccines, kids are in school, teenagers aren't pregnant, that's kind of the backbone of the health care system." But preventive care is also about things that happen outside a doctor's office. Recent research has found that the risk of heart disease, even for those with family histories, decreases by half if people don't smoke, get exercise at least once a week, eat healthy food and aren't obese (even if they are overweight). But some of those are hard things to accomplish in the Black Belt. As was the case when Peterson was growing up in Thomaston, people must often travel long distances to reach a grocery store, which makes it hard to get fresh produce. As in many rural areas, there are few sidewalks in the Black Belt, and the hot weather during parts of the year is not conducive to exercise outside anyway. Waits counts lack of exercise as among the biggest barriers to health for people in the region.

Trust and Access

And there are more intimate problems as well, such as communication between doctors and patients. "It definitely takes time, being a white doctor, for a black resident to trust you. To some extent that's true everywhere, but it's lengthier and deeper here," Waits said. "Some of it relates to relatively recent medical ethics."

Waits was referring to the notorious Tuskegee syphilis experiments, in which researchers deprived a group of black men with syphilis of treatment for some 40 years, until 1972, in order to study the progression of the disease. But that's not the only cause of a documented lack of trust of medical professionals among African-Americans. Trust is a hard - to-measure but important aspect of how researchers gauge the ability of a provider to address a patient's needs once she reaches a facility.

African-Americans are more likely to report being treated with disrespect by a doctor and are less likely to be health literate than whites, which can make it difficult to understand prescription drug labels or complete medical forms. And research shows that African-Americans do receive different treatment than whites. The 2015 National Healthcare Quality and Disparities Report from the Agency for Health care Research and Quality found that black Americans received worse care than whites on 41 percent of health care measures.

A doctor such as Remona Peterson, who is African-American and comes from the community, is likely to be a key part of the solution here. She said her whole reason for going to medical school was to take her intimate understanding of the area where her family has lived for more than a century and use it to improve her community's health. The issues of trust and access hit home: Peterson remembers an aunt who was hypertensive and uninsured. She didn't think any of the local doctors would see her, so she received little in the way of treatment. She had a stroke and died at age 54.

In some ways, Peterson's winding path from straight- A student to rural doctor could help her adjust to working in such a challenging environment. Peterson hopes that she'll be able to communicate more effectively with her patients and that they'll trust that she cares. She also hopes she'll be better at understanding their needs beyond physical and mental health. That could include making sure they have transportation to appointments or remembering to prescribe generic drugs people can afford. All of this could go a long way toward improving access to care. "If you grow up in this, you know what it's like," she said.

Peterson alternated between concern and excitement about what's ahead. "I worry if I'm going to be good enough for them, for my people. I want to do my best; I want to be good enough." She also described her ideal rural practice: a bus that can go and get patients, an office with a nutritionist, an exercise program, community health educators. She has high hopes for the future.

"There's so much we could do in the Black Belt; I don't even know where to start. I know what I can do as a doctor," Peterson said, "but it's going to take more than just me. It's going to take a team of people who want to see the community change and get better." Peterson will soon be part of that team. She will join the staff of the Greene County Health System on July 24.

Ms. Sewell. I have placed this article in the record before and I will continue to do so because I think it is important that we address solutions acknowledging that healthcare is not a one-size-fits-all, but acknowledging that there are differences between urban areas, suburban areas, and rural areas.

I agree with Dr. Waits, who likes HSAs, and I am not an opponent to it. I just don't see it as a cure-all. I don't even see it as helping to address the underlying problems, which is the escalating cost of healthcare, when so many of my constituents can't afford to save in their 401(k), let alone save money through health savings accounts.

So in the 11 counties of my district, the average median household income is $28,000. And I know that you, Ms. Dietel, talked about median income being around $58,000. Well, my district is way below that.

And here is the rub. I am a proud product of my district. I am a product of my district that through education had other opportunities, and I had a chance to work in a really great law firm that offered me a health savings account, which I did participate in.

But the reality is that the majority of folks that I represent in my district can't make that same choice. And in fact, I get a little upset when I think that people view folks that I represent as not being personally responsible for their healthcare because they can't afford to save in these health savings accounts.

It is just the flip of that, frankly. These are people who are struggling every day to put food on the table for their children, to provide better opportunities for their children, who want preventive medicine, who want better access to healthcare. So many of them don't even have transportation to the nearest healthcare provider.

And I would agree with my colleague, Earl Blumenauer, that we do need to talk about infrastructure financing, because telehealth can't come to parts of my district in rural Alabama because we don't have broadband.

So there are real issues about healthcare that we in this committee address. And in fact I am on the bill that Mr. Kelly and Mr. Blumenauer, the bipartisan bill about improving HSAs, the health savings accounts. So to the extent that we are going to have them, I do believe we need to have reform.

I guess my question is to you, Ms. Glied. I want to make sure that we are addressing the real problem, which is access to healthcare, the rising cost of healthcare, and making sure that we in America, the land of the plenty, actually do have healthcare that can reach every part of America irrespective of one's ability to pay.

Ms. Glied. I couldn't agree with you more. I think your point is exactly correct. We need to think about how to direct our tax dollars to the people who are going to need that the most.

As we think about reforming HSAs, I think what that should help us to think about is, as Representative Blumenauer pointed out, making the design of these changes as targeted as possible to exactly the problems we think that we need to address. So, for example, perhaps chronic disease management.

But opening them up a lot just means sending a lot of tax dollars to people who really don't have these problems, and that means tax dollars that are not available to provide care to people who do.

Ms. Sewell. Yeah. And, listen, I would love if you, Ms. Dietel, would work with my staff to figure out the statistics in my district in terms of median income and their ability to use HSAs.

Like I said, I am not against that. I just think that at the end of the day, there are whole host of reasons that go into the rising cost of healthcare. And I don't think that health savings accounts actually gets to the problem really, which is access to healthcare and the cost of healthcare for folks that I represent.

Will you commit to helping my –

Ms. Dietel. Absolutely. In fact, we had a meeting with your staff yesterday.

Ms. Sewell. I know. But I think your numbers are contradictory to what –

Ms. Dietel. And we are going to follow up with your specific information. We discussed ways to expand it. For example, Healthy Indiana would be a great solution for your district as well.

Ms. Sewell. Okay. Thank you.

Chairman Roskam. Thank you.

Look, on behalf of the subcommittee, thank you for your testimony today. Just to put this in a little bit of a context for you as witnesses, this subcommittee has taken on a task of inquiring of healthcare providers on a bipartisan basis on what are the regulations that don't make any sense and what makes things more expensive for you to deliver healthcare?

And we have done a series of roundtable discussions. We have gotten 500 submissions from healthcare providers. And it has been a fascinating discussion. It is one that has sort of transcended some of the normal political dialogue on healthcare. So it is not as if we are only evaluating HSAs as a remedy here, but there is very much a tapestry that we are trying to put together.

So I just have a number of questions in closing.

Dr. Glied, I am getting a mixed message from you. So on the one hand, you have been harshly critical of HSAs. And on the other hand, you are a little bit complimentary of them. Is the system better off without HSAs, in your view? Or what is the role?

Ms. Glied. The question is not whether the system is better off. On the whole, HSAs are going to make the healthcare system spend a little bit more money than it would if there were high-deductible plans without HSAs. And a concern is that making HSAs more available actually just increases the enthusiasm for high-deductible plans, which I think are bad for a lot of people.

The challenge is not about HSAs, though. The challenge is really whether we want to give tax breaks to HSAs. That is really the question. People could have HSAs anyway. They can on their own open savings account.

Chairman Roskam. Right. For sure. Okay.

Ms. Glied. The question is, where should the tax money go?

Chairman Roskam. Right. Okay. I got it. That is clear to me.

So the enthusiasm for high-deductible plans, Mr. Eyles, doesn't come in a vacuum. It is not as if people just say, "Oh, I want to spend more money on the front end." What is the benefit of this? So in other words, the context is a lower premium, right?

Mr. Eyles. Oh, absolutely. I mean, it is all about tradeoffs. We can either have lower premiums and maybe have a consumer-directed health plan with an HSA attached to it, or we could have plans that are much more expensive that might cover more, as Mr. Ramthun was talking about, a higher actuarial value. It is all about tradeoffs.

And what we are supportive of is making sure that people have access to some of these tax-deferred mechanisms to offset the impact of some of the deductibles that perhaps they are facing and do it in a way that also provides greater flexibility, greater choice, greater convenience for consumers who want to spend their own healthcare dollars.

Chairman Roskam. So it is connected to a benefit. It is a level of discipline and so forth that yields a benefit in terms of a lower premium?

Mr. Eyles. That is right. I mean, as we have look at the premiums for a typical HSA plan or eligible plan versus, say, a traditional PPO, it is probably about 10 to 15 percent less being in an HSA plan.

And we are talking about in the individual market or in the small group market, there is one common risk pool, at least in terms of how ratings get set, but these plans can be less expensive and they also provide benefits to consumers who can use those dollars.

Chairman Roskam. I understand.

Mr. Ramthun, in your opening testimony and your statement, you spoke about actuarial value. Can you, first of all, describe what that is? And then that 80 percent figure, did you pull that out of the air?

But first of all, describe what it is that you are proposing.

Mr. Ramthun. So if you think of actuarial value as an overall measure, like the metal tiers in the Affordable Care Act offer –

Chairman Roskam. The value of a policy.

Mr. Ramthun. Value of the policy. How rich of benefit coverage is there? Does it pay 70 percent of the cost on average, 80 percent, 60 percent? We know those as Bronze, Silver and Gold Plans today.

What it avoids is some of the details of these plan design features and saying it must look like this, it must look like that in order to qualify, which is what we have today.

So the design gives you more flexibility for plans to address all of the concerns that have been raised here at the committee level and do it in a way where the choice can be made by the consumer, "Do I want to be in that plan or do I want a different flavor of that?"

I don't think we want to make necessarily every plan, a plan that covers 100 percent of your costs, should those people have HSAs too? Probably not. They are not available to those individuals in the marketplace today. Probably not the best place for us to start. But this could go a long way to freeing up some of the challenges that everybody has mentioned today, more on a laundry list of challenges.

Chairman Roskam. It is sort of interesting because there is a theme that is consistent with this regulatory relief project, and the theme is this: When you pose the question on regulatory relief, you invite a different discussion. The new discussion is that one person's burdensome regulation is another person's patient protection.

That is a rational discussion. We can navigate through that based on good science and good data and so forth. And what you are suggesting here is you can dial these attributes up, and you can dial them back.

But to observe HSAs in a vacuum, only in the context of high-deductible, is to not recognize the benefit of a lower premium and what a lower premium means to families across the spectrum.

Okay, Ms. Dietel, I have a question for you. Listening to Dr. Glied, my interpretation of her criticism was this really benefits people that don't need a benefit. This benefits wealthier people. And yet, you are communicating $56,100 income level. That strikes me as modest, in the great scheme of things.

Can you reconcile that? Who is it that you are finding is using these plans and benefiting from these plans? Because from my point of view, that is not uber wealth. I mean, that is not even particularly affluent, $56,100. Can you just walk us through that?

Ms. Dietel. Sure. So we came up with the household income data by appending the data with geocoded data, much like mortgage lenders do. And so I think it is statistically valid.

We have actually met with the Joint Committee on Taxation, IRS, Treasury folks, OMB, and NEC on the same data, and I think that we are working hard – and Roy and I have been on this effort, too – to try and help understand the differences between IRS data and our data that is prevalent in the marketplace.

I think the other thing we have seen is that as we have studied the data, particularly over the last 10 years with the rapid expansion of high-deductible health plans that are HSA qualified, I think that we have seen those average incomes, median household incomes come down rapidly.

I remember first walking the Hill in 2009, and we were sitting at more like $88,000 for a median household income for an HSA account holder. So I think that it is much more of a rank-and-file plan.

I also think one important point to remember is that the average deductible of any health plan in America is higher than the statutory minimum deductible right now, and that is in my written testimony.

And so high-deductible health plans have inherent problems, much of which I agree with Ms. Glied. I think that health savings accounts, though, are important particularly since the Affordable Care Act is built on the employer system, 170 million Americans get their coverage through the employer market.

And if on the ACA side we believe that a family of four making upwards of $105,000 needs premium subsidies and cost-sharing support, why would we remove the only safety net or the only tool that working Americans have through these consumer-directed benefit accounts to provide them with help for these out-of-pocket costs.

Much work to do. We will be happy to continue to help.

Chairman Roskam. Are you communicating some of that information to the Joint Committee on Taxation and so forth?

Ms. Dietel. Yes, sir.

Chairman Roskam. Because you are on the front lines. It is no surprise to us to hear that the counters here. These entities that are charged with giving us information are behind the curve. I mean, they just don't have access to the same type of data.

So are you sharing that information now with Joint Committee on Taxation and so forth?

Ms. Dietel. Yes, sir.

Chairman Roskam. Okay. That is helpful, because I think that will help the debate all the way around.

Do you have an opinion about this notion of expanding first-dollar coverage and its impact on premiums? What happens if first-dollar coverage is expanded?

Mr. Eyles.

Mr. Eyles. We haven't done specific actuarial modeling, but I think the types of services that we are talking about would not have a significant impact on premiums. We are really talking about high value services that we think over time would enable people to stay healthier and probably have lower trend over time.

But we are not talking about all of a sudden opening up the floodgates to all types of treatments and services to be covered pre-deductible. That would have a significant impact on premiums. We are talking really much more targeted efforts.

Chairman Roskam. Okay. I think that this has been a very fruitful discussion, in my view. And I am sensing some body language from my friend from Michigan.

Am I sensing any body language? The gentleman is recognized.

Mr. Levin. Thanks. I am sorry I missed most of the earlier discussion. I was at the Bobby Kennedy 50-year memorial. But in a sense I arrived, and it is more or less the same old debate, the same old assumptions. And I think we need to talk through these assumptions.

Mr. Kelly talks about healthcare, but it is different than any other product. And the knowledge of people about healthcare is more complicated than it is buying lots of other things.

I think people have to take better care of themselves. That is very true. But other countries have learned, and I think this country has learned, that purchasing healthcare is a much deeper challenge and the ability to be knowledgeable is more difficult. And we have worked hard to get prevention into healthcare, sometimes over the opposition of people on the other side.

When you eliminate the original mandate and you have HSAs more and more prevalent, you are essentially going to raise the cost of insurance for everybody else. The healthier people are going to buy the policies that take more risk because they are younger in most cases and they think it is fine.

And we were headed more and more in that direction and we decided we needed to do what every other country did, and that is to really increasingly make insurance available. And there have been efforts to tear it down. And so far those efforts are a major cause of the increase in premiums, if not the only.

So I want to enter into the record, if I might, two things. First of all, my opening statement.

Chairman Roskam. Without objection.

RANKING MEMBER SANDY LEVIN, OPENING STATEMENT, HEALTH SUBCOMMITTEE HEARING, WEDNESDAY, JUNE 6, 2018

In 2010, President Obama signed into law the Affordable Care Act, and over the past eight years our health care system has undergone a historic transformation. The uninsured rate among the nonelderly has dropped by more than 40 percent. Health plans must now cover all Essential Health Benefits, including preventive care, prescription drugs, and substance use treatment. And 130 million Americans with preexisting conditions can no longer be discriminated against or denied coverage by insurers.

If all those who have benefited from the ACA formed a single line, it would nearly wrap twice around the globe.

Despite this remarkable progress, Republicans continue to undermine the implementation of the law. Last fall, the Administration slashed the advertising budget for the Open Enrollment period and cut funding for Navigator organizations that help consumers sign up for coverage.

More recently, CMS issued several regulations that weaken consumer protections and could destabilize the individual market by moving healthier enrollees into short-term policies and Association Health Plans.

Republican Members of this Subcommittee have actively supported this sabotage while calling for repeal of the law and a reversal of the historic gains made over the past eight years.

In place of the comprehensive coverage provided through the ACA, Republicans propose to move consumers into high-deductible plans paired with expanded health savings accounts. This is a prominent feature of

Speaker Ryan's Better Way agenda, the Senate's Graham-Cassidy bill, and the American Health Care Act that was marked up by the Ways and Means Committee last year. Each proposal fails to meaningfully address the documented shortcomings of high-deductible plans and health savings accounts.

First, and foremost, is the issue of affordability of care. High-deductible health plans live up to their name. According to the Kaiser Family Foundation, the average deductible for a family plan is more than $4,600, while nearly a quarter of families in face a deductible of $6,000 or more. These are staggering amounts, particularly in light of the fact that the majority of households do not have enough savings to cover even a $1,000 emergency.

Faced with unexpected health expenses, an HSA paired with a high-deductible plan is often just a fig leaf. Not all employers contribute to HSAs, leaving millions of workers entirely responsible for funding their account - which many cannot afford to do. Moreover, among those middle-class Americans who are able to contribute to these accounts, their lower marginal rate makes this benefit worth less to them than it is to the wealthy.

There is also little evidence that high-deductible plans have any impact in controlling health care cost growth. Rather than making consumers smarter shoppers, the lack of price transparency and higher out-of-pocket costs simply force many to go without the care they need. This is particularly harmful to lower income consumers, who are more likely to end up in the emergency room or require inpatient hospitalizations.

In short, despite the promises made by their proponents, high-deductible plans and health savings accounts are not a substitute for comprehensive coverage. Instead of focusing on this narrow issue, which has proven inadequate for meeting the needs of consumers, this Subcommittee should take a different focus and join the effort to expand access to affordable, quality health care to all Americans through the ACA.

Mr. Levin. Secondly, a document that has been prepared by the Ways and Means staff that shows in terms of HSAs 81 percent of the tax benefit goes to the top 8.7 percent of account holders. And so when you talk about averages, it is important that we really look at the impact in terms of the taxation and the tax benefits.

And I think the concern of most of us is not opposition to HSAs under any circumstance, but the essential movement towards more when steps are being taken to provide healthcare insurance to fewer. That is what has happened in this country. People who were covered by ACA, now it is more difficult for them to access it.

So we had this remarkable increase in the percentage of people having healthcare insurance in this country, remarkable. Not good enough. But we are working in the opposite direction now.

And so I think we need to have this full, forthright discussion, and essentially we have passed tax health legislation, and there hasn't been enough adequate discussion about where this country is going.

So I want to enter this into the record.

Chairman Roskam. Without objection.

CONGRESS OF THE UNITED STATES JOINT COMMITTEE ON TAXATION

June 6, 2018

Memorandum

To:

From: Thomas A. Barthold

Subject: Follow-up on the distribution of HSA and FSA contributions

On June 5, 2018 we responded to your request for information about the distribution of Flexible Spending Account ("FSA") contribution and Health Savings Account ("HSA") contributions. In our response, we provided a distribution table showing, separately by income class, the number of returns and dollar value of contributions to FSAs, employer contributions to HSAs, and HSAs contributions claimed as a deduction against income.

As a follow-up, you requested that we also include the tax value of these contributions. We determined the tax value of contributions in a manner similar to the method we use to estimate tax expenditures. In the case of FSAs and employer contributions, we calculated the income tax value of such contributions by adding the contributions to wages on the return and computed the resulting change in income tax liability. In the case of HSAs claimed as a deduction, we repealed the deduction and computed the resulting change in income tax liability. These estimates are not revenue estimates as we did not account for possibly behavioral responses by taxpayers or their employers. The estimates are for tax year 2015.

The table we provided to you on June 5 showed, by income class, the number of returns and dollar amounts of FSA contributions, HSA contributions claimed as a deduction on Fann 1040, and employer contributions to HSA accounts. The attached table is the same as the previous table except that we added columns for the estimated income tax value of these contributions.

Ms. Levin. And I am sorry I missed earlier, but the staff will bring me up to date.

And, Mr. Chairman, I think, at the very least what these hearings do indicate is the need to really dig more deeply. And I just want to join Mr. Blumenauer. Though you don't see, most people, the relationship between infrastructure and healthcare, they are somewhat interconnected. And I just hope that this committee will step up to the plate when it comes to both healthcare reform further and infrastructure.

With that, I yield back having 1 second left. Chairman Roskam. Thank you very much.

I think that there are many themes that bring us together. There are differences that you hear among us. I think the good news for you, Mr. Levin, is that I think Ms. Dietel's information is going to update the Joint Committee on Taxation, which is what I assume that document was built on that was just made part of the record.

Table 3. Distributions of employer contributions to health savings accounts, and employee contributions to flexible spending accounts (FSA) form 1040 deduction for health savings account (HAS) contributions, counts of returns, dollar value of contributions, and the income tax value of contributions, in tax year 2015

	Employee Contributions to FSAs			Employer Contributions to HSAs			Deduction for HSA Contributions		
Income Class(1)	Number of Returns	Dollar Value Contributions	Tax Expenditure Value (2)	Number of Returns	Dollar Value Contributions	Tax Expenditure Value (Z)	Number of Returns	Dollar Value Contributions	Tax Expenditure Value (3)
	Millions	$Billions	$Billions	Millions	$Billions	$Billions	Millions	$Billions	$Billions
Less than $10,000	0.6	0.4	(5)	14)	(5)	(S)	(4)	(5)	(5)
$10,000 to $20,000	0.2	0.2	(5)	0.1	0.1	(5)	(4)	(5)	(5)
$20,000 to $30,000	0.4	0.4	(5)	0.3	0 .2	(5)	(4}	0.1	(5)
$30,000 to $40,000	0.4	0.4	0.1	0.5	0.5	0.1	0.1	0.1	(5)
$40,000 to $50,000	0.6	0.6	0.1	0.6	0.7	0.1	0.1	0.1	(5)
$50,000 to $75,000	1.6	1.7	0.3	1.4	2.0	0.4	0.2	0.4	0.1
$75,000 to $100,000	1.5	1.9	0.4	1.1	2.0	0.4	0.2	0.5	0. 1
$100,000 to $200,000	3.7	5.4	1.3	2.7	7.3	1.7	0.4	1.3	0.3
$200,000 to $500,000	1.5	2.5	0.8	1.2	4.6	1.4	0.3	1.2	0.4
$500,000 to $1,000,000	0.2	0.3	0.1	0.1	0.7	0.3	0.1	0.4	0.1 -
$1,000,000 and over	0.1	0.1	0.1	0.1	0.3	0.1	(4)	0.2	0.1
Total, All Taxpayers	10.9	14.0	3.1	8.1	18.3	4.5	1.4	4.3	1.1

Source: Joint Committee on Taxation Detail may not add to total due to rounding.

(1) The income concept used to place tax returns into income categories is adjusted gross income (AGI) plus: [1] tax-exempt Interest, [21employer contributions for health plans and life insurance, [3) employer share of FICA tax, [4] worker's compensation, [51nontaxable Social Security benefits, [61insurance value of Medicare benefits. [7] alternative minimum tax preference items, [8] individual share of business taxes, and [9) excluded income of U.S. citizens living abroad.

(2) Calculated by adding the contribution amount to wages. No other behavioral adjustments assumed. (3) Calculated by repealing the deduction. No other behavioral adjustments assumed. (4) Less than 50,000. (5) less than $50 million.

So the proof will either be there or it won't. But my sense is she is the canary in the coal mine and I think is going to have a much better sense, notwithstanding the admonitions from Dr. Glied right now, but I think that is actually true.

I think that there is a real opportunity for us to work together on this and the notion that people have just more – you know, an insurance card – I will go back to Mr. Kelly's point – an insurance card alone does not yield coverage. And I think what we are all trying to do is to get around these areas so that more people are more satisfied, with better coverage and more choices, than ever before.

And so I know that there is a number of other folks that will have some input on this. I ask unanimous consent to submit a statement for the record from the Alliance of Health Care Sharing Ministries. Without objection, that is ordered.

Chairman Roskam. And, again, members are reminded that they have got 2 weeks to submit written questions that can be answered later in writing. And those questions and answers would be made part of the formal record.

Again, thank you to the witnesses for your time today. The committee stands adjourned.

[Whereupon, at 12:41 p.m., the subcommittee was adjourned.]

MEMBER QUESTIONS FOR THE RECORD

Thank you, Mr. Chairman, and thank you to all of you for being here this morning.

Since the inception of Flexible Spending Arrangements (FSAs) and Health Savings Accounts (HSAs), millions of Americans each year were using these and other similar tax-preferred health accounts to help reduce their annual healthcare spending. However, this consumer access changed with the passage of the Affordable Care Act.

Consumers are now required to obtain a prescription for over-the-counter medications in order to be eligible for reimbursement under these accounts. This change, which went into effect January 1, 2011, severely limits the ability of millions of American families to use funds set aside in their FSAs and HSAs to purchase over-the-counter products, such as those for pain management, smoking cessation, and cold and allergy medications.

Over-the-counter medications are often the frontline treatment for many common illnesses or for maintenance of chronic diseases and should be treated as medically reimbursable healthcare therapies, just as prescription medications are. A study conducted by Booz and Co. found that over-the-counter medicines save the U.S. healthcare system $102 billion every year, through cost savings associated with over-the- counter medicines and avoided visits to the doctor. Restricting consumers' ability to be reimbursed under FSAs and other tax-preferred accounts imposes an unfair cost-increase on individuals and families who may already be struggling financially. That's why I've re-introduced common-sense legislation with Mr. Kind to restore this benefit, H.R. 394 the Restoring Access to Medication Act, and I urge my colleagues to join us in passing this legislation once again.

According to an April 2014 study by Nielsen, 75 percent of Americans support changing the law to grant over-the-counter medications tax-preference once again. In fact, the Health Choices Coalition, representing physicians, dentists, consumers, retailers, manufacturers, pharmacies, pharmacists, patients, insurers, and employers large and small are all in support of restoration of this benefit on behalf of millions of Americans.

1) Americans are being asked to fund more of their health care expenses through higher deductibles and copays, so I believe it's more important than ever that cost- effective over-the-counter medicines are treated the same as other eligible medical expenses in tax-preferred health care accounts. I don't know *why we should be making it harder* for Americans to use their own pre-tax dollars to purchase these every-day health care products. So, Mr. Eyles, shouldn't Congress be making it easier for people to access these safe and effective over-the-counter medicines?

2) And on that point, as I have often said, so many Kansas communities face the challenges that come with accessing rural health care. Mr. Ramthun, do you believe that it makes good policy-sense to require patients, especially rural patients, to seek a doctor's prescription in order to be able to use their tax-advantaged accounts for medicines that are available over the counter?

Thank you and I yield back.

STATEMENT FROM THE CONSUMER HEALTHCARE PRODUCTS ASSOCIATION, COMMITTEE ON WAYS AND MEANS, HEARING ON LOWERING COSTS AND EXPANDING ACCESS TO HEALTH CARE THROUGH CONSUMER-DIRECTED HEALTH PLANS, WEDNESDAY, JUNE 6, 2018

The Consumer Healthcare Products Association (CHPA) appreciates the opportunity to provide the following statement regarding the Committee on Ways and Means hearing on "Lowering Costs and Expanding Access to Health Care through Consumer-Directed Health Plans."

Since 1881, CHPA has served as the industry association representing leading manufacturers and marketers of over-the-counter (OTC) medicines in the United States. CHPA member companies produce the vast majority of OTC medicines in our country and provide millions of Americans with safe, effective, and affordable therapies. The availability of self-care treatment options saves money, reduces burdens on the healthcare system, and keeps consumers active and productive.

OTC and prescription medications are regulated for safety and effectiveness by the U.S. Food and Drug Administration (FDA). It is especially important to recognize that OTC medicines are often the frontline or only treatment available to some consumers for many common illnesses or for maintenance of chronic diseases. While not only are OTC medicines the accessible option for both consumers and the U.S. healthcare system, a study conducted by Booz and Co. found that OTC medicines save the U.S. healthcare system $102 billion every year, and for every dollar spent on OTC medications in the U.S., the healthcare system saves $6 to $7.

However, OTC medicine eligibility in tax-preferred accounts was removed in 2011 as one of the first-implemented provisions of the Affordable Care Act (ACA).

Restricting consumers' ability to utilize their own FSAs and HSAs and other tax-preferred accounts imposes an unfair cost increase on individuals and families at a time when many are struggling financially.

Americans are being asked to fund more of their healthcare expenses through higher deductibles and copays, so it's more important than ever that cost-effective OTC medicines are treated the same as other eligible medical expenses in tax-preferred healthcare accounts.

Restoring OTC eligibility under FSAs and HSAs will help the more than 50 million consumers who use these accounts and who are looking to take greater ownership of their own health through responsible self-care.

Further, this provision contradicts the intent of healthcare reform by increasing expenditures in the healthcare system such as increased physician visits to obtain a prescription for OTC medications. It imposes a medically unnecessary tax and treatment burden on patients, encumbers overworked physicians with unnecessary office visits, all without advancing the quality of healthcare overall. According to a study conducted by the American Osteopathic Association, 65 percent of osteopathic physicians surveyed have been asked by their patients to write prescriptions for OTCs, while 95 percent of osteopaths surveyed believe those patients could have self-treated successfully.

CHPA has been leading a broad national coalition – the Health Choices Coalition (HCC) – advocating for restoration of this important consumer benefit. The HCC includes consumer advocates, policymakers, physicians, dentists, retailers, pharmacies, pharmacists, insurers, drug manufacturers, and various employers.

This Congress, bipartisan, bicameral legislation that would restore the ability of consumers to use their tax-preferred FSAs and HSAs to purchase OTC medicines has been introduced. The legislation, "Restoring Access to Medication Act (RAMA) of 2017" (H.R. 394 and S. 85), was introduced in the Senate by Senators Pat Roberts (R-Kan.) and Heidi Heitkamp (D-N.D.), and in the U.S. House by Representatives Lynn Jenkins (R-Kan.) and Ron Kind (D-Wis.). This comes on the heels of a vote in the previous Congress, that restored this benefit, enabling Americans to utilize these tax-favored health accounts to purchase over-the-counter medications, which passed the House of Representatives by a vote of 243-164.

CHPA appreciates the opportunity to share our views on this important matter and looks forward to continuing to work with the Committee and with the Congress to restore this benefit on behalf of the millions of Americans who rely on OTC medicines for everyday ailments.

Congressman Earl Blumenauer Statement for the Record before the Ways and Means, Subcommittee on Health, June 6, 2018

Mr. Chairman, while I appreciate the subcommittee's attention to improving our healthcare system, I am struck that this is another missed opportunity to address one of the most pressing economic, health, and safety issues of today: our nation's infrastructure. The Ways and Means Committee has held 393 hearings since 2011, but only devoted five minutes to infrastructure- five minutes of testimony in nearly seven and a half years. In every American community, there are deep concerns about the state of our roads, bridges, transit, water systems, ports, airpotts, and broadband connectivity. Today, one in five miles of highwa y pavement is in poor condition, and two of five urban highway miles are congested,[58] forcing our constituents to spend more money fixing their car and more time sitting in traffic rather than being with their loved ones.

---

[58] American Society of Civil Engineers, 2017 Infrastructure Report Card- Roads.

This Committee's inaction on infrastructure has also resulted in degrading health and safety outcomes. In 2016 alone, 37,461 Americans were killed in fatal automo bile crashes and more than two million Americans are routinely injured in traffic accidents every year[59] – costing our economy over $63 billion from the cost medical care and lost productivity[60]. The health impacts of long commutes and traffic congestion are also clear: phys ical inacti vity, increased risk of depression and anxiety, chronic stress, and higher blood pressure. The consequences of the disrepair of our water infrastructure are also well-documented, with communities like Flint, Michigan forced to take drastic measures to protect the health and well-being of their citizens.

There is no area of greater political consensus than on the need to rebuild and renew America. Since 2012, 31 states of political backgrounds have raised transportation revenues, demonstrating the broad, bipartisan support for infrastructure funding and finance. On Capitol Hill, countless stakeholder groups from across the political spectrum stand ready and willing to testify on the importance of infrastructure investment; a list of some of these groups is attached. It is past time that the Ways and Means Committee takes an active role on providing the leadership and courage to rebuild and renew Ame1ica. I look forward to pattnering with my colleagues to get this done.

Supporters of Renewing the Federal Partnership on Infrastructure

- AAA
- American Association of State Highway and Transportation Officials (AASHTO)
- American Bus Association

[59] National HighwayTraffic Safety Administr ation, "USDOT Releases 2016 Fatal Traffic Crash Data," October 6, 2017.

[60] Center for Disease Control a nd Prevention, Web-basedlnjwy Statistics Query and Reporting System, 2013.

- American Coal Ash Association
- American Concrete and Pavement Association
- American Concrete Pipe Association
- American Council of Engineering Companies (ACEC)
- American Highway Users Alliance
- American Iron and Steel Institute
- American Public Transportation Association (APTA)
- American Road & Transportation Builders Association (ARTBA)
- American Society of Civil Engineers (ASCE)
- American Subcontractors Association
- American Traffic Safety Services Administration (ATSSA)
- American Trucking Associations
- Associated General Contractors of America (AGC)
- Associated Equipment Distributors
- Association for Commuter Transportation
- Association of Equipment Manufacturers
- Asphalt Emulsion Manufacturers Association
- Asphalt Recycling & Reclaiming Association
- Commercial Vehicle Safety Alliance
- Concrete Reinforcing Steel Institute
- Geosynthetic Materials Association
- Getting America to Work Coalition
- Highway Materials Group
- International Slurry Surfacing Association
- International Association of Bridge, Structural, Ornamental and Reinforcing Iron Workers
- International Brotherhood of Teamsters
- International Union of Operating Engineers
- ITS America
- Laborers-Employers Cooperation and Education Trust
- Laborers International Union of North America
- League of American Bicyclists

- Los Angeles County Metropolitan Transportation Authority
- National Asphalt Pavement Association
- National Association of Surety Bond Producers
- National Association of Truck Stop Operators
- National Electrical Contractors Association
- National Ready Mixed Concrete Association
- National Steel Bridge Alliance
- National Stone, Sand, and Gravel Association
- National Utility Contractors Association
- Owner Operator Independent Drivers Association (OOIDA)
- Portland Cement Association
- Precast/Pre-stressed Concrete Institute
- Railroad Cooperation and Education Trust
- The Road Information Program
- Transportation for America
- United Brotherhood of Carpenters and Joiners of America
- United Parcel Service (UPS)
- U.S. Chamber of Commerce

Public Submissions for the Record

Statement of the American Hospital Association, before the Committee on Ways and Means of the U.S. House of Representatives, "Hearing on Lowering Costs and Expanding Access to Health Care through Consumer- Directed Health Plans," June 6, 2018

On behalf of our nearly 5,000 member hospitals, health systems and other health care organizations (approximately 100 of which sponsor health plans), and 43,000 individual members, the American Hospital

Association (AHA) appreciates the opportunity to submit for the record our comments on consumer-directed health plans and their relationship to lowering costs and expanding access to care for patients.

Health care affordability is a significant challenge for many individuals and families, and we appreciate policymakers' exploration of potential solutions to address this issue. This hearing will consider whether consumer-directed health plans can be a part of the solution. The AHA defines consumer-directed health plans as those plans that pair a health savings account (HSA, usually tax-advantaged) with a high-deductible health plan (HDHP). Patients use funds from the HSA to pay for most services until a minimum deductible has been reached; the HDHP covers some limited preventive care, as well as catastrophic costs. These plans generally offer lower premiums than more conventional insurance products and, therefore, may appeal to more cost- conscious consumers or those who expect to have fewer health care needs.

Consumer-directed health plans may be an appropriate form of coverage for some individuals, including those who have high health care literacy and sufficient means to fund their HSAs or otherwise cover higher upfront costs. However, the AHA is concerned about the ability of these plans to lower costs and expand access to care for individuals who may not be aware of the limitations of such coverage and who do not have the means to fund their HSAs or otherwise pay for initial care out of pocket.

Hospitals and health systems report that increased enrollment in HDHPs over the past several years has *reduced* access to care and subjected patients to costs they cannot afford. In addition, patients enrolled in HDHPs appear to delay care until they have reached their deductible or are in an emergency situation, which could lead to poorer health outcomes.

While we recognize that these types of health plans are intended to promote consumer engagement in their health, we are concerned that the evidence does not currently support this assertion. Hospitals and health systems report that many patients in HDHPs do not understand their coverage. Instead of being active purchasers, patients are often surprised to learn what their health plan does and does not cover when they are at the point of care, and this information may not contribute to shopping for the best value but rather to opting not to pursue care at all.

The impacts identified above may vary if an entity besides the patient, such as an employer, funds the HSA. However, employer funding of HSAs is on the decline, and this is not an option for the millions of consumers who rely on the individual market. According to United Benefit Advisors, "The average employer contribution to an HSA is $474 for a single employee (down percent from 2015 and 17.6 percent from five years ago) and $801 for a family (down 9.2 percent from last year and 13.7 percent from five years ago)."[61] These figures account for approximately a third of what the minimum deductible must be for a plan to qualify as an HDHP. Therefore, even when employers do contribute to an HSA, patients retain the bulk of the financial responsibility.

Improving Access and Reducing the Cost of Coverage

Without addressing the underlying cost of care, insurance benefit designs like HDHPs and HSAs simply "shuffle the deck chairs." In other words, HDHPs do not necessarily reduce the right costs (e.g., low-value care or medically unnecessary care), they shift responsibility for upfront costs from one entity to another – first from the payer to the consumer and then to providers in the form of bad debt. We encourage Congress to pursue actions that will help improve the cost of coverage without putting access to care at risk, including:

1) Addressing the underlying drivers of high cost, such as the unsustainable growth in prescription drug prices; duplicative, unnecessary and potentially harmful regulatory and administrative burden; and high rates of chronic disease; and

[61] United Benefit Advisors, "Special Report: How Health Savings Accounts Measure Up," May 2017.

2) Promoting enrollment in comprehensive health care coverage to share costs across the broadest population possible, including through stabilizing the health insurance marketplaces.

We recognize that HDHPs coupled with HSAs will continue to be an attractive option for some individuals. We encourage Congress to improve on these by re-examining the services that insurers may offer pre-deductible or which may be covered by funds in an HSA. For example, we specifically support expanding insurers' ability to cover care for chronic conditions pre-deductible. This change would help remove financial barriers patients may face while managing their health. In addition, we strongly encourage the federal and state governments, employers and other payers to coordinate on a robust consumer education campaign on the importance of having health coverage and how to use it. The campaign should specifically address how different types of health plans may affect both premiums and upfront, out-of-pocket costs.

Conclusion

We appreciate the opportunity to provide these comments and support the Committee's efforts and attention to examining the issues concerning access to care and the affordability of coverage. We are deeply committed to working with Congress, the Administration, and other health care stakeholders to ensure that all individuals and families have the health care coverage they need to reach their highest potential for health.

June 4, 2018

The Honorable Peter Roskam
Chair, House Ways and Means
Subcommittee on Health
2246 Rayburn House Office Building
Washington, D.C. 20515

The Honorable Sander Levin
Ranking Member, House Ways and Means
Subcommittee on Health
1236 Longworth House Office Building
Washington, D.C. 20515

Dear Chairman Roskam and Ranking Member Levin:

On behalf of the American Association of Oral and Maxillofacial Surgeons (AAOMS), the professional organization that represents 9,500 oral and maxillofacial surgeons (OMSs) in the United States, I would like to thank you for your leadership in identifying ways to lower healthcare costs by holding the June 6th Subcommittee hearing titled, "Lowering Costs and Expanding Access to Health Care through Consumer-Directed Health Plans." The issue is important to OMSs since many of our patients often rely on consumer-directed health plans, such as Flexible Spending Accounts (FSAs), to help them afford the treatment they need.

Current restrictions stemming from the ACA established a federal cap on FSA contributions at $2,500 – with an annual inflation adjustment – which was half of the $5,000 limit that most employers allowed prior to the adoption of the ACA. Out-of-pocket costs for medical insurance alone easily exceed the current $2,650 annual FSA cap. With the rise in cost of deductibles, co-pays and prescription drug medications, Americans are paying more for their healthcare. According to the 2017 Milliman Medical Index, consumers spent an average of $4,535 for out-of-pocket healthcare expenses in 2017.[62] This is significantly more than what consumers are able to save through FSAs.

FSAs also help patients afford dental care. Oral health is increasingly recognized as being tied to a patient's overall health and well-being; however, health insurance does not cover most dental procedures and many Americans do not have access to dental insurance. Even for those who do, dental insurance only covers a fraction of the cost of many common and necessary dental procedures, like dental implants,

[62] Girod C, Hart S, Weltz S. 2017 Milliman Medical Index. Milliman, Inc. 2017: 3-15.

orthodontia, root canals or extractions of abscessed teeth. As a result, families rely often on the tax-free savings from FSAs in order to help them save for these types of procedures. With the existing restrictions on FSA contributions, some patients are forced to forgo necessary dental care.

The Responsible Additions and Increases to Sustain Employee Health Benefits Act of 2017, or RAISE Act (HR 1215), would provide relief to families by raising the cap to $5,000 and allowing families with more than two dependents to set aside an additional $500 beyond the savings cap for each dependent. Finally, it would help families prepare for expected and unanticipated healthcare costs by carrying over unused funds and eliminating the IRS's onerous "use it or lose it rule."

AAOMS encourages the Subcommittee to take up the RAISE Act (HR 1215) as it evaluates ways to lower healthcare costs through consumer-directed plans. FSAs enable consumers to make better healthcare decisions and control their healthcare costs. We welcome an opportunity to discuss this issue in greater detail and work with you and your Committee to increase the contribution limits to FSAs.

Sincerely,

Brett L. Ferguson, DDS, FACS
AAOMS President

Statement for the Record, House Way and Means Health Subcommittee Hearing, "Lowering Costs and Expanding Access to Health Care through Consumer-Directed Health Plans," June 6, 2018

The American Council of Life Insurers (ACLI) is pleased to submit the following statement for the record for the House Ways and Means Committee hearing "Lowering Costs and Expanding Access to Health Care through Consumer-Directed Health Plans" held June 6, 2018. Specifically, we are writing in support of Section 2 of H.R. 5138, the Bipartisan HSA

Improvement Act of 2018, co-sponsored by Rep. Mike Kelly and Rep. Earl Blumenauer. ACLI strongly supports including the provisions of Section 2 in any health savings account (HSA) legislation moving through Congress.

ACLI advocates on behalf of approximately 290 member companies dedicated to providing products and services that contribute to consumers' financial and retirement security. ACLI members represent 95 percent of industry assets, 93 percent of life insurance premiums, and 98 percent of annuity considerations in the United States. 75 million families depend on our members' life insurance, annuities, retirement plans, long-term care insurance, disability income insurance and reinsurance products. Taking into account additional products including dental, vision and other supplemental benefits, ACLI members provide financial protection to 90 million American families.

Some of the products provided to consumers by ACLI member companies include "excepted benefits" as described in Internal Revenue Code Section 9832(c). "Excepted benefits" are generally defined as those benefits that are not considered "health insurance coverage" or are limited in scope and offered separately from health insurance. The "excepted benefits" which ACLI member companies provide are in addition to health insurance to fill gaps in primary coverage and are not a replacement for primary health insurance. Under IRC Section 9832(c), "excepted benefits" are listed specifically and include disability income insurance, long-term care insurance, limited scope dental and vision benefits if offered separately from a major medical plan, coverage for specific disease or illness, hospital indemnity or other fixed indemnity insurance, and similar supplemental coverage if offered as a separate policy.

Current law governing HSAs, IRC Section 223(c), uses a limited list of supplemental products in its definition of "permitted insurance" and should be updated to conform with HIPAA's definition of "excepted benefits" to avoid unnecessary and burdensome confusion in the marketplace. Such dissimilarity currently creates a strong disincentive to an employee's purchase of certain supplemental benefits if they use an HSA in combination with a High Deductible Health Plan because the purchase of such insurance protection disqualifies an employee from being eligible for the HSA. As a result, the current law definition of "permitted insurance" limits consumer choice and the ability of the employee to craft an individualized package of optimum financial protection to add to their primary major medical coverage.

Section 2 of H.R. 5138, represents a long-overdue update that will appropriately modernize IRC section 223(c) to conform the HSA "permitted insurance" definition to the HIPAA "excepted benefits" definition – the same definition that is also included in the Public Health Services Act, the Employment Retirement Income Security Act and the Patient Protection and Affordable Care Act. This "excepted benefits" update will also provide clarity to employers who are not always sure if a supplemental benefit they would like to provide to their employees is allowed to be offered alongside an HSA.

As the Committee considers ways to improve and expand the use of consumer-driven health plans to expand coverage and lower health care costs, we respectfully urge you to pass H.R. 5138.

AFLAC, INC., WRITTEN STATEMENT FOR THE RECORD FOR "LOWERING COSTS AND EXPANDING ACCESS TO HEALTH CARE THROUGH CONSUMER-DIRECTED HEALTH PLANS," COMMITTEE ON WAYS AND MEANS, HEALTH SUBCOMMITTEE, UNITED STATES HOUSE OF REPRESENTATIVES, JUNE 6, 2018

We are writing in support of legislation to expand the use and availability of health savings accounts and high deductible health plans.

In particular, we support section 2 of H.R. 5138, and section 1 of H.R. 6128, which represent a long-overdue technical correction to the 1996 HIPAA law for "excepted benefits" insurance. This change will conform the HSA "permitted insurance" text to the "excepted benefits" text that is used in ERISA, the Public Health Service Act, and other provisions of the Internal Revenue Code that lists "excepted benefits" insurance coverage.

These "excepted benefit" insurance products are not purchased with HSA funds. The HSA law permits a policyholder to have some supplemental insurance products in addition to the HSA-High Deductible Health Plan. As a result, this technical correction would not take away any amounts available in the HSA to be used for necessary "qualified medical expenses."

In addition, we respectfully ask the committee to consider simply striking inconsistent excepted benefits references in current law subparagraphs (B) and (C). These coverages are also included in section 9832(c).

Our concern is that leaving current subparagraphs (B) and (C) would maintain inconsistent statutory text. We also support language to address concerns about excepted benefit coverage that is not appropriate for high deductible health plans. Within the context of the excepted benefits provision in both H.R. 5138 and H.R. 6128 these two changes would be drafted as follows:

(a) In General. – Paragraph (3) of section 223(c) of the Internal Revenue Code of 1986 is amended by –

(1) striking subparagraphs (B) and (C), and

(2) inserting the following new subparagraph:

> "(B) insurance consisting of coverage of excepted benefits described in section 9832(c) other than supplemental coverage provided to coverage under a group health plan described in subparagraph (4).

We thank the committee for its effort with respect to this bipartisan legislation, and for considering our suggestions to clarify these provisions.

CORPORATE HEALTH CARE COALITION

June 22, 2018

The Honorable Kevin Brady
Chairman
U.S. House Ways & Means Committee

The Honorable Richard Neal
Ranking Member
U.S. House Ways & Means Committee

The Honorable Peter Roskam
Chairman, Subcommittee on Health
U.S. House Ways & Means Committee

The Honorable Sander Levin
Ranking Member, Subcommittee on Health
U.S. House Ways & Means Committee

Dear Messrs. Brady, Roskam, Neal and Levin:

The Corporate Health Care Coalition (CHCC) is pleased to comment on the hearing recently held by the House Ways and Means Health Subcommittee, entitled "Lowering Costs and Expanding Access to Health Care through Consumer-Directed Health Plans." With 22 million Americans currently enrolled in Health Savings Accounts (HSAs), it is clear that HSAs play an increasingly valuable role in America's health care system.

CHCC is comprised of companies from varying industries that compete in the global marketplace and sponsor health plans for the benefit of our employees and other beneficiaries.

Collectively, CHCC member companies provide health benefits for more than 4 million Americans across every state in the nation. CHCC companies are committed to providing access to affordable, quality health care benefits and HSAs are a valuable source of health care coverage for many of our beneficiaries.

CHCC supports federal efforts to modernize HSAs to reflect advances in employee benefits by allowing greater access to primary care and chronic disease management, wellness offerings, and streamlining the conversion from a Medical Savings Account, Flexible Spending Arrangement or Health Retirement Arrangement to an HSA. Specifically, CHCC supports H.R. 5138, the Bipartisan HSA Improvement Act of 2018 (the Kelly-Blumenauer bill) and H.R. 365, the Primary Care Enhancement Act of 2017 (the Paulsen-Blumenauer bill).

H.R. 5138, the Bipartisan HSA Improvement Act, allows employers to cover health services such as those provided at onsite medical clinics and through telemedicine. H.R. 365, the Primary Care Enhancement Act, clarifies that direct primary care, which is a coordinated, high- functioning care model proven to prevent emergency room visits and hospitalizations, is not a health plan. By doing so, the bill would allow those contributing to an HSA and enrolled in a high-deductible health plan, to also enroll in a direct primary care arrangement.

Employers are leading the way in health care innovation by promoting payment for value, incentivizing employees to seek care from high performing providers, encouraging wellness and prevention, and exploring new care models and provider partnerships to improve quality, affordability and accountability. We urge Congress to act to pass H.R. 5138 and H.R. 365 to bolster the value and effectiveness of HSAs as a critical part of our nation's health care infrastructure.

Sincerely,

Kate Hull

Executive Director, Corporate Health Care Coalition

Statement of Support for the Personal Health Investment Today (PHIT) Act to Be Included in HSA Health Care Package

Tuesday June 19th, 2018

Congressman Brian Fitzpatrick

I am pleased to be a supporter of the Personal Health Investment Today (PHIT) Act which would allow a medical care tax deduction for up to $1,000 ($2,000 for a joint return or a head of household) of qualified sports and fitness expenses per year.

The PHIT Act would provide incentives for adults and children to pursue healthy lifestyle choices. Equipping Americans to get fit in this way would not only improve general health and well-being but would also mitigate against healthcare costs related to preventable chronic diseases.

As healthcare expenses in the U.S. continue to rise, the PHIT Act would help build a healthcare system that prioritizes prevention. The World Health Organization reports that every $1 of investment in physical activity in the U.S. leads to $3.20 in medical costs saving. For these reasons, I believe any effort or immediate plans to improve or reduce the long-term costs of healthcare in this country should include the PHIT Act as it is a forward-thinking, citizen-focused, incentives-driven and economically beneficial piece of legislation.

PatientRightsAdvocate.org 1188 Centre Street

Newton, MA 02459

June 20, 2018

Chairman Peter Roskam

Dear Chairman Roskam:

We are pleased that the House Ways and Means Health Subcommittee is exploring policy solutions to lower the costs of health care services and expand access to care through Health Savings Accounts (HSAs). Thank you for the opportunity to comment on this important issue.

PatientRightsAdvocate.org believes that patients should have total net price transparency prior to care and real-time access to their comprehensive electronic health information, as soon as the data are recorded.

HSAs Alone Cannot Solve the Health Care Cost Problem

We appreciate the role that HSAs can play to empower patients; however, patients cannot make rational economic choices when the prices of health care are in a black box. Patients should have total price transparency for their health care services, including both the negotiated price and out-of- pocket costs, prior to care. This information will enable patients to shop for the most cost-effective treatment, budget accordingly, and efficiently leverage tools such as HSAs. Patients will then be empowered to manage their own care and will not receive any surprise bills.

We Need Total Price Transparency to Ensure a Competitive Market

With true total price transparency, all parties on the payment side of a transaction (patient, employer, health plan, pharmacies, and government) will have easily accessible and downloadable information about the price of health care services prior to services rendered. Requiring this transparency is a common sense solution that will have a ripple effect across the health care industry. Enabling a transparent, efficient, truly competitive market will drastically lower costs and ultimately improve the care of our citizens. Thank you again for the opportunity to comment. Sincerely,

Kara Grasso
President, PatientRightsAdvocate.org

June 14th, 2018

The Honorable Kevin Brady
Chairman
House Ways & Means Committee

The Honorable Richard E. Neal
Ranking Member
House Ways & Means Committee

The Honorable Peter Roskam
Chairman, Subcommittee on Health
House Ways & Means Committee

The Honorable Sander Levin
Ranking Member, Subcommittee on Health
House Ways & Means Committee

Dear Chairmen and Ranking Members:

The American Council on Exercise would like to thank you for the opportunity to submit written testimony for the Ways & Means Health Subcommittee's June 6 hearing on Lowering Healthcare Costs through Consumer- Directed Health Plans. The American Council on Exercise (ACE) is a self-funded 501C-3 nonprofit organization that works to improve physical-activity levels in America by educating and certifying exercise professionals and health coaches, publishing independent original research, convening experts on physical activity and health, working directly with community groups, and advocating for policies to get people from all walks of life moving.

Medical flexible spending accounts (FSAs) have been served as a popular addition to many employer's benefits packages for many years. While health savings accounts (HSAs) are a newer addition to consumer driven healthcare options, they have grown steadily since their inception and are now considered by many a mainstay, if not the future, of the commercial health insurance market. As you are undoubtedly aware, both FSAs and HSAs allow individuals and families to utilize pre-tax dollars to pay for medical expenses from prescription meds, to routine doctor visits to elective procedures such as Lasik eye surgery. The missing category for allowable expenses under current law is physical activity.

Research has shown that physical inactivity increases the risk of developing numerous preventable health conditions that contribute greatly to our skyrocketing healthcare costs. Research has also demonstrated that engaging in regular physical activity contributes to an individual's overall feeling of well-being which is keenly important when considering mental health.

We believe that a consumer-directed health plan must include options for physical activity. It is a cornerstone of a more prevention-centered way of caring for the health and wellness of our nation's people. Reps. Jason Smith and Ron Kind introduced HR1267, the Personal Health Investment Today Act (PHIT) early in the Congress that would make physical activity expenses allowable under FSAs and HSAs. PHIT has wide bi-partisan support with 134 co-sponsors, almost evenly split between the parties. The same language has been included in several larger bills as well including the recent Bipartisan HSA Improvement Act (H.R. 5138) that was introduced by Reps Mike Kelly and Earl Blumenauer.

We were pleased to hear Rep. Kelly discuss the the need for individuals to do "preventative maintenance" in terms of their health while stressing the importance of prevention to the health and economy of our country. Only 21.6% of children and youth ages 6 participate in at least one hour of physical activity per day as recommended in the Physical Activity Guidelines for Americans while 80% of American adults do not meet the government's national physical activity recommendations for aerobic and muscle strengthening. Healthcare policies to date have considered physical activity expenses a luxury, but science has shown exercise to be just as vital to preventing chronic disease as medicines are to treating illness.

Allowing use of consumer driven health plans for physical activity would allow families to use a portion of their pre-tax dollars to help pay for their children's sports fees as well as dance classes, martial arts, etc. It would allow individuals and families to use those same dollars to take group exercise classes, join a fitness center or otherwise engage in structured physical activity.

Overwhelmingly, studies show that physical activity plays an important role in preventing and managing chronic diseases-the same diseases that are responsible for 86 percent of our nation's healthcare costs. The American Council on Exercise hopes that as the committee considers their options around consumer driven health plans that they consider physical activity a key component and include language such as the PHIT Act.

Best Regards,

Sheila Franklin
Director of Government Relations
American Council on Exercise

Cynthia A. Fisher
WaterRev LLC

June 20, 2018
Chairman Peter Roskam

Dear Chairman Roskam:

Thank you for your efforts to give more consumers access to tax-favored savings accounts, including Health Savings Accounts (HSAs). I appreciate the opportunity to submit comments for consideration by the House Ways and Means Health Subcommittee. HSAs are an important tool to help reduce the burden of health care costs on patients. However, a tax-favored account has limited effectiveness since patients rarely know upfront the prices they are going to pay for their medical care and services. Imagine taking a pre-funded debit card to a restaurant, only to receive a menu of food options with no prices.

Patients Need Total Net Price Transparency

Instead of focusing on HSAs, Congress and CMS should mandate that patients receive total net price transparency prior to care. Patients should be informed of the lowest net negotiated price, competitive pricing from other providers or health plans, and out-of-pocket costs for their care before they receive any treatment or medical service. They should also be notified if a potential doctor is out-of- network and the out-of-network charges, and where they could receive complete services in-network. There should be no surprise billing.

Transparency Will Enable a Competitive Market

Patients and employers should be able to shop for their care on their mobile devices by having access to total net price transparency, free of charge. Like in a restaurant, patients should be able to see the prices, order from the menu, and the bill should match the care they received. Then and only then will an HSA benefit the patient. Patients, employers, and our government should have full visibility into what the health plans are covering, and we should be able to view comparative pricing among health plans. Patients should also have the choice to continue with their health plan throughout their lifetime.

Patients also Need Access to Their Comprehensive Electronic Health Information

This includes but is not limited to, discharge summaries, lab and radiology results, prescription orders, images, and physician notes Patients should have access as soon as the data are recorded, with regular, automatic updates thereafter. In virtually every other industry, you can receive and share results through mobile apps immediately as they are available. The same should be true with our health care information as soon as it becomes digital.

Patients Should Have Control of Their HSAs

Currently, third party vendors manage HSAs and profit on the float until the monies are spent on health care services. If these are my tax-favored dollars, I should receive the interest, dividends, and gains. Similar to the successful 529 plans, I should be able to park my HSA in the index funds of my choice, have transparency into fees, choose where the monies are held and how they are invested.

Unused HSA Dollars Should Be Transferrable

Any unused monies at year-end should not be lost; they still belong to the patient/consumer. The balance should be able to be transferred into the consumer's retirement account, to another person in need, or to next year's HSA. They also should be inheritable to family or others upon death.

Thank you again for the opportunity to comment on the improvements needed to HSAs.

Sincerely,

Cynthia A. Fisher
Managing Director, WaterRev, LLC
Founder, Former CEO, ViaCord, Inc.
Founder, Former President, ViaCell, Inc.

International Health, Racquet & Sportsclub Association

June 12, 2018

The Honorable Kevin Brady
Chairman
House Ways & Means Committee

The Honorable Richard E. Neal
Ranking Member
House Ways & Means Committee

The Honorable Peter Roskam
Chairman, Subcommittee on Health
House Ways & Means Committee

The Honorable Sander Levin
Ranking Member, Subcommittee on Health
House Ways & Means Committee

Dear Chairmen and Ranking Members:

The International Health, Racquet & Sportsclub Association (IHRSA) would like to thank you for the opportunity to submit this written testimony as part of the Ways & Means Health Subcommittee's June 6 hearing on Consumer-Directed Health Plans such as Health Savings Accounts (HSAs) and Flexible Spending Accounts (FSAs). IHRSA is the leading trade association representing the private health and fitness industry, with over 7,000 members in 74 countries. Our members are committed to policy initiatives aimed at promoting exercise, preventing disease and improving the health of all Americans, hence our interest in consumer-directed health plans.

HSAs and FSAs are becoming increasingly important parts of the American healthcare landscape and have experienced significant growth in the commercial insurance market since they were created.

Through these accounts, individuals and families are able to pay for doctors' visits and other medical treatments with pre-tax dollars thereby helping to ease the financial burden when Americans pay for medical treatment once they are sick. However, current law offers no tax benefit to help individuals and families take steps to prevent illness in the first place.

This at a time when the Centers for Disease Control and Prevention (CDC) estimates that close to 70 percent of adults suffer from some form of chronic disease, with lack of physical activity standing as one of the top four preventable causes of these diseases. At the same time, CDC also estimates that roughly 79 percent of Americans fail to meet even the most basic recommendations for aerobic and strength training activity.

In the context of this disturbing reality and the Subcommittee's June 6 hearing, IHRSA strongly believes that the existing consumer-directed health plan system should be expanded to provide for more disease prevention by allowing expenses for exercise programs and related equipment to be payable out of HSA/FSA monies. Several members of the House have introduced legislation over the years to address this issue by expanding HSAs and FSAs to allow exercise expenses to qualify for pre-tax distributions. Such legislation includes H.R. 1267, the Personal Health Investment Today Act (PHIT), introduced by Reps. Jason Smith and Ron Kind and a more comprehensive package of reforms (H.R. 5138) introduced by Reps. Mike Kelly and Earl Blumenauer.

In fact, during the hearing on June 6, Rep. Kelly warned that "if we don't get people healthy early on, we're in big trouble." Clearly, Mr. Kelly recognizes the need for policy initiatives like the PHIT bill which would help make the healthy choice the easy choice.

If these provisions are enacted, it would give parents the opportunity to pay for their children's soccer league fees out of their tax deferred plans. They could join a fitness center and pay for the membership fees with pre-tax dollars or they could purchase a home gym to help them fight the onset of obesity, a primary risk factor for contracting any one of several chronic diseases which are currently fueling the frightening increase in our national healthcare expenditures.

Health experts agree that regular physical activity substantially reduces the risk and symptoms of numerous diseases and medical conditions and is associated with fewer hospitalizations, physicians' visits, and medications, resulting in lower healthcare costs. Expanding tax incentives to include programs of physical activity would lower financial barriers to exercise and help more people get the levels of activity they need to improve their fitness and lower healthcare costs for all Americans.

Given the healthcare crisis we are facing in this country today, IHRSA and its members strongly believe that creative solutions are necessary to improve the nation's physical fitness. As the Ways & Means Committee considers future adjustments to the consumer-directed health plan system, we urge you to take the next step and move forward to enact legislation that would make expenses for exercise payable with pre-tax dollars, such as the PHIT Act mentioned above.

IHRSA and its members stand ready to help advance these kinds of initiatives aimed at improving the health of all Americans. Please let us know how we can work together to achieve this critical objective.

Sincerely,

Joe Moore
President
International Health, Racquet & Sportsclub Association
cc: Members of the House Ways and Means Committee

Healthcare Leadership Council
June 6, 2018

The Honorable Peter Roskam
Chairman
Subcommittee on Health
Committee on Ways and Means
United States House of Representatives
Washington, D.C. 20515

Dear Chairman Roskam:

Thank you for holding a hearing on consumer-directed health plans. The Healthcare Leadership Council (HLC) appreciates the opportunity to share its thoughts with you on this important issue.

HLC is a coalition of chief executives from all disciplines within American healthcare. It is the exclusive forum for the nation's healthcare leaders to jointly develop policies, plans, and programs to achieve their vision of a 21st century healthcare system that makes affordable, high-quality care accessible to all Americans. Members of HLC – hospitals, academic health centers, health plans, pharmaceutical companies, medical device manufacturers, laboratories, biotech firms, health product distributors, post-acute care providers, and information technology companies – advocate for measures to increase the quality and efficiency of healthcare through a patient-centered approach.

To give consumers choice and flexibility in their healthcare, HLC strongly believes that the Subcommittee should support the expanded use of consumer-directed health plans. Restoring options and increasing the flexibility of health savings accounts (HSAs), as well as repealing the limitations on contributions to HSAs and flexible spending accounts (FSAs), will provide consumers with better tools to manage their funds and cover healthcare expenses.

HLC is pleased to support H.R. 5138, the "Bipartisan HSA Improvement Act." Introduced by Subcommittee members Mike Kelly and Earl Blumenauer, this important legislation would assist the more than 20 million Americans who have an HSA. The bill would modernize HSA plans by:

- Allowing pre-deductible coverage of services at onsite employee clinics and retail health clinics;
- Enabling pre-deductible coverage for services and medications that manage chronic health conditions;
- Clarifying that employers can offer excepted benefits like telehealth and second opinion services to employees with an HSA; and
- Making technical changes to correct the definition of dependents, streamline FSA conversion, and fix the prohibition on spouse usage of HSAs.

Additionally, H.R. 5138 would permit the use of HSA dollars for wellness benefits and physical activity expenses. Chronic disease prevention is an essential component of healthcare. Many of these illnesses, including obesity and diabetes, are caused by modifiable health risk behaviors such as poor nutrition and a lack of physical activity. If not prevented, these diseases and their complications raise healthcare costs.

Americans need access to comprehensive and evidence-based wellness and physical activity programs that assist them in making healthy choices and preventing these diseases. "The Bipartisan HSA Improvement Act" would expand this access and make these programs more affordable.

HLC asks the Subcommittee to support H.R. 5138 and include it in its consideration of consumer-directed health plans.

Sincerely,

Mary R. Grealy, President

Statement for the Record, U.S. House Ways and Means Committee, Subcommittee on Health, Hearing: "Lowering Costs and Expanding Access to Health Care through Consumer-Directed Health Plans," June 6, 2018

Chairman Roskam, Ranking Member Levin and Members of the Committee:

The Partnership for Employer-Sponsored Coverage appreciates the Committee holding this hearing today to highlight the importance of consumer-directed health products such as health savings accounts (HSAs) and welcomes the opportunity to endorse the *Bipartisan HSA Improvement Act, H.R. 5138*.

The Partnership for Employer-Sponsored Coverage is a newly-formed advocacy alliance of employment-based organizations and trade associations representing businesses of all sizes and the over 178 million American workers and their families who rely on employer-sponsored coverage every day. The Partnership is committed to working to ensure that employer-sponsored coverage is strengthened and remains a viable, affordable option for decades to come.

Employer-sponsored coverage has been the backbone of our nation's health system for over seven decades. Employers of all sizes contribute vast resources to their employees and families through the employer-sponsored system.

As the payer of coverage, employers have a vested interest in health care quality, value, and system viability. Employers have been on the leading edge of health delivery innovation and modeling for decades.

In the 15 years since the Ways and Means Committee created HSAs under the Medicare Prescription Drug, Improvement, and Modernization Act (P.L. 108-173), utilization has grown tremendously among employers of all sizes and in the small group and individual insurance markets. Currently, more than 20 million Americans are covered by an HSA with a high-deductible health plan (HDHP) through employer-sponsored coverage or coverage in an insurance Exchange.

Over the last decade, employers of various sizes have either transitioned from a traditional preferred provider organization (PPO)-based system to an HSA with a HDHP or offered this arrangement as an option during open enrollment to provide employees with more cost-effective health coverage and consumer choice. As health costs have increased for working Americans and employers alike, an HSA coupled with a HDHP has become a more viable option to enable thousands of businesses to continue offering employment-based health coverage.

As the Ways and Means Committee and your colleagues in Congress explore ways to improve the usefulness of an HSA with a HDHP, the Partnership for Employer-Sponsored Coverage urges enactment of the *Bipartisan HSA Improvement Act, H.R. 5138*. There has been an increase in the variety of benefits offerings sponsored by employers since HSAs were created in 2003.

Unfortunately, our nation's federal tax code has not kept pace with the advances in employer benefits offerings.

The Bipartisan HSA Improvement Act, which is sponsored by your colleagues Representatives Mike Kelly (R-PA), Earl Blumenauer (D-OR), Erik Paulsen (R-MN), Ron Kind (D-WI), and Terri Sewell (D-AL), aligns the HSA rules in the Code with the evolving and improving benefits offerings sponsored by employers.

Among other provisions, H.R. 5138: allows for first dollar coverage of services for chronic care and disease management; provides for the use of services at employer on-site and retail clinics; and enables employees to use an HSA for wellness benefits including gym memberships.

The Partnership for Employer-Sponsored Coverage looks forward to working with you and your colleagues in Congress in a bipartisan manner to enact H.R. 5138 and other commonsense reforms to strengthen and improve our nation's employment-based health system, which serves as the safety net for over 178 million Americans every day.

Partnership for Employer-Sponsored Coverage Members:

- American Hotel & Lodging Association
- American Staffing Association
- American Rental Association
- Associated Builders and Contractors, Inc.
- Auto Care Association
- HR Policy Association
- International Franchise Association
- National Association of Health Underwriters
- National Association of Wholesaler-Distributors
- National Restaurant Association
- National Retail Federation
- Retail Industry Leaders Association
- Society of American Florists
- Society for Human Resource Management

Statement of Pat LaFontaine of National Hockey League, on Youth Sports Benefits and Barriers to Sports Participation, House Ways and Means Subcommittee on Health, Wednesday, June 6, 2017

Thank you Chairman Roskam, Ranking Member Levin and Members of the Committee, for holding a hearing on HSA reform and allowing me to provide input on this very important subject.

I currently serve the National Hockey League as Vice President of Hockey Development for the Social Impact, Growth Initiatives and Legislative Affairs unit. During my playing career, I had the privilege to represent the United States on the 1984 Olympic Men's Ice Hockey Team and spent 15 seasons in the State of New York, with the NHL's New York Islanders, Buffalo Sabres and New York Rangers. In 2003, I was inducted into the Hockey Hall of Fame and in 2017 was humbled to be recognized as one of the NHL's Top 100 Players of all-time. The sport of hockey has given me so much, far beyond awards, medals and scoring records. The game provided me foundational elements for life: values, friendships, life skills and more. In my current role, I am dedicated to growing and developing the game of hockey in a way that ensures our sport delivers the best possible family experience, so that all youth have access to the same benefits of the game that I enjoyed.

I commend the committee for holding this hearing and exploring ways to improve our current healthcare system. While there are many good ideas to advance the performance of our system and reduce costs, the most sustainable way to reduce health spending in America is to improve our collective health. Healthy habits are formed when we are young; youth sports is a vital element of American culture, is essential to establishing healthy lifestyles long-term and a key component to solving our health care challenges.

I will focus my comments today on the health benefits of active lifestyles and how the PHIT Act will help families reduce barriers to entry for our youngest generation.

In 2017, the National Hockey League and National Hockey League Players' Association took a leadership role in this space when it unveiled hockey's Declaration of Principles a set of commonly shared beliefs and a commitment to advance policies, programs and initiatives that inspire key stakeholders to refocus on the true value the sport provides and the importance of access and opportunity for all. Hockey participation offers families value beyond making an individual a better player or even a better athlete. The game of hockey is a powerful platform for participants to build character, foster positive values, develop important life skills and encourage a lifetime of healthy behaviors. We know that physical activity – like ice hockey, roller hockey and street hockey – is important for a healthy body, mind and spirit. It is the goal of the broader hockey community – backed by 17 global stakeholders – to bring the benefits of sports to all American families.

The youth sports culture in America has changed. Accessible, community-based recreational youth sports opportunities – such as house ice hockey programs – have been replaced by a pay-for-play, race to the top mentality manifesting in elite-focused programming. The size of a family's bank account now plays an outsized role in youth sports. In hockey, this market change flies in the face of objective data: less than 2% of hockey participants will receive a college scholarship, and less than a fraction of a percentage will play in a professional league. This is not unique to the game of hockey, and has contributed to a higher rate of burn-out, injury and drop-out of youth sports participation at critical ages across the board. This effort is too important to the future health of our nation for us to stand idly by, both physically and fiscally. The World Health Organization reported that a one-dollar investment in physical activity in the U.S. will result in a $3.20 reduction in future health costs – this is real prevention! Youth sports activity has an important role to play in disease prevention and driving down pressure on our healthcare system.

The Personal Health Investment Today (PHIT) Act, legislation introduced by House Ways & Means Members Jason Smith and Ron Kind and supported by 63 Republicans and 70 Democrats in the House, including half the members of the Ways & Means Committee, will help lower the cost of active lifestyles by giving consumers the option of using pre-tax medical dollars to pay for activity expenses. PHIT will encourage consumers to invest in active, healthy lifestyles. This includes children's team registration fees, pay-to-play fees in schools, activity-based park programs, access fees, tournaments, camps and clinics. PHIT does not increase caps on pre-tax accounts and limits reimbursements to "expenses exclusively intended for sole purpose of participating in a physical activity." PHIT is not about encouraging materialism, as the purchasing of items like basketball shoes, yoga pants or jerseys as apparel and footwear are specifically and rightfully excluded as eligible expenses. PHIT is drafted to help with legitimate expenses incurred by families seeking to live and provide healthy, active lifestyles. Our society has changed and active lifestyles require an investment that previous generations did not incur. Congress can help Americans lower the cost of active, healthy lifestyles by passing the PHIT Act.

Congress would be smart to take this action as it would help directly respond to very important issues faced by our country and our communities, from rising health care costs, to national security, to gangs, drugs and violence.

CDC reports indicate that 20 percent of children in the U.S. are obese and 70 percent of the American adult population is overweight or obese; this is a very real epidemic, and we are heading for a deluge of chronic disease and exponential reliance on the healthcare system, as the sedentary population requires more expensive and consistent medical attention and procedures. . Fortunately, the CDC has also recognized that active lifestyles reduce the incidence of Type 2 Diabetes, cardiovascular disease, dementia, depression, anxiety and many types of cancer – lending significant support to the value the PHIT Act provides to the health care system.

Today, seven-in-ten new military recruits are unfit to serve; the poor health of our youth threatens our military readiness and national security. Youth athletic participation has an important role to play in the development of our future force – physically, emotionally and cognitively. The strength of our military thrives on the quality of its people. Youth sports produces better athletes, better leaders and better teammates, who develop an understanding of rules, ethics and respect. These values and skills are transferable and extremely valuable characteristics to find in future military recruits.

Congress has done a great deal of work on the opioid crisis – along with efforts on gangs and violence – yet we have failed to recognize and include youth sports activity as part of the solution. This is true despite numerous studies by the National Institutes of Health on the critical role of activity in treating opioid addiction. Physical activity releases endorphins and dopamine, combating one's need to find that stimulus elsewhere. Moreover, the community created by athletics provides an important space for our youth to invest their time in something positive, and build relationships and trust with people from all backgrounds. Significant behavioral research has confirmed that youth sports is an important outlet and support mechanism for children and families, offering us all opportunities to make better choices, ones that lead away from gangs, violence and drugs. In addition to the positive humanitarian effect, investing in youth athletics helps treat root causes of these problems, offering a sustainable reduction in costs associated with these issues.

I thank you for your time and this opportunity to discuss the important role of physical activity in addressing our national health care concerns. I encourage Congress to promote active, healthy lifestyles – and this begins with the passing of the PHIT Act.

I am available to answer any questions, to further elaborate on any contents in this letter or to speak in more depth about the vital role of athletic participation in this country.

June 4, 2018

The Honorable Mike Kelly
U.S. House of Representatives

The Honorable Earl Blumenauer
U.S. House of Representatives

Dear Representatives Kelly and Blumenauer:

On behalf of the Retail Industry Leaders Association (RILA), I am writing to thank you for introducing the *Bipartisan HSA Improvement Act of 2018* (H.R. 5138). RILA, the trade association of the world's largest and most innovative retail companies, product manufacturers, and service suppliers, is committed to ensuring employer-sponsored health care remains a viable option for the 170 million Americans receiving coverage today.

Over the last several years, many RILA member companies have moved away from traditional fee-for-service plan offerings to a system coupling a health savings account (HSA) with a high- deductible health plan (HDHP). The transition is guided by retailer's innovative approach to customizing benefit designs and creating health plans that best meet the needs of their employees and families. HSAs with a HDHP help to control rapidly increasing health costs, which is crucial to the long-term well-being of employer-sponsored coverage.

The *Bipartisan HSA Improvement Act* creates more flexibility and value for retail employees who utilize HSAs. It allows for employees to access onsite or retail primary care clinics, pre- deductible coverage for chronic disease management, and opportunities to use HSAs for fitness or wellness activities. Providing more usable benefits under an HSA could lead to decreases in health care spending, minimize hospitalization or inpatient stays, and better overall health.

RILA also appreciates the Ways and Means Subcommittee on Health for convening a hearing on June 6, 2018, on *"Lowering Costs and Expanding Access to Health Care through Consumer-Directed Health Plans."* This represents an important first-step to examine how consumer-directed health care products, such as HSAs, can improve outcomes, incentivize preventative and primary care, and enhance the health of the retail employees throughout the U.S. RILA member companies will gladly provide any assistance needed to the committee's work as potential HSA related policies move through the legislative process.

As the U.S health care system continues to evolve, we believe unique benefit design packages with HSAs will become an increasingly important component of a healthy workforce. Again, thank you for introducing H.R. 5138. RILA looks forward to working with you and your colleagues in Congress in a bipartisan manner to enact this legislation.

Sincerely,

Jennifer Safavian
Executive Vice President, Government Affairs

cc: The Honorable Kevin Brady
The Honorable Peter Roskam
The Honorable Richard Neal
The Honorable Sander Levin

STATEMENT OF THE SPORTS AND FITNESS INDUSTRY ASSOCIATION, ON THE POWER OF PHYSICAL ACTIVITY IN PREVENTING CHRONIC DISEASE, HOUSE WAYS AND MEANS SUBCOMMITTEE ON HEALTH, WEDNESDAY, JUNE 6, 2018

Mr. Chairman, Ranking Member Levin and members of the Committee thank you for holding this hearing on HSA reform. The healthcare system has gone through great changes since these accounts were created, and now they need modification to best serve consumers in today's healthcare marketplace. Medical science supports the importance of prevention and wellness as consumers take a more proactive role in their healthcare and employers offer incentives to live a healthy lifestyle. In fact, the CDC has called physical activity a "wonder drug" that can prevent chronic disease, including heart disease, type II diabetes, dementia, depression, anxiety and many types of cancer. As more and more evidence has emerged, regarding the extensive health benefits of activity, some people have taken steps to be more active. However, according to the Physical Activity Council, 82 million Americans are still completely sedentary. The best way to combat this problem and reduce healthcare spending is by encouraging a healthier, more active population.

The Sports & Fitness Industry Association (SFIA) was established in 1906, and for the past 111 years, our mission has been to promote personal health and well-being and the clinical evidence that links physical activity with reduced healthcare costs.

The Personal Health Investment Today (PHIT) Act (H.R. 1267) encourages activity by lowering the cost of various activity fees, such as youth sports registrations, pay-to-play fees in schools, gym memberships, fitness & yoga classes and personal trainers. The PHIT Act would also cover any equipment that is exclusively used for activity. Currently, 133 House members (63R-70D), including 19 who serve on the Ways & Means Committee, agree on the need for a physical activity incentive and signed on as co-sponsors of PHIT. As the Committee considers legislation designed to update the usefulness of health savings accounts, we encourage you to include PHIT in any HSA package.

Last month, SFIA joined with multiple business groups in a letter describing the trends taking place in today's workplace around increased enrollment and consumer demands for more flexible healthcare benefits.

The message is clear - A culture change is needed to improve health in America. This includes a multi-faceted approach toward reducing obesity rates, teaching our youth the importance of physical fitness and helping seniors manage their chronic conditions with the help of exercise. We have the least active generation of children in history. According to the Robert Wood Johnson Foundation, it has been reported that inactive children are six times more likely to be inactive parents with inactive children. If the inactivity rate among children today remains the same, Johns Hopkins University estimates the economic impact to be $2.7 trillion dollars over the course of their lifetimes. In short, the future of health in America looks bleak and is headed in the wrong direction.

The CDC identifies "lack of resources" as one of the main reasons for inactivity. To overcome poor health in the U.S. and soaring healthcare expenses, we need to help parents with the costs of children's activity to get them started on the right path. This lifestyle change will provide the foundation for children to remain active throughout their life. With PHIT, we are promoting an investment in health to encourage this exact culture change, starting with young people.

We have put forth a strong effort in creating a fully-encompassing, yet focused piece of legislation that optimizes user benefits. The PHIT Act has been tightly drafted to focus on just the necessities: allowance for the "sole purpose of physical fitness." The PHIT Act explicitly excludes footwear and apparel and instead, only permits expenditures for equipment, gym memberships, and the other aforementioned items described earlier. Moreover, the legislation explicitly caps equipment expenses at $250 for individual purchases. This will help parents support the ever increasing drain taking place in today's "pay-to-play" youth sports leagues and after school activities.

SFIA strongly supports an expansion of eligible expenses for HSAs to make these accounts more consumer-friendly. HSAs continue to grow as the healthcare marketplace evolves, and now more people rely on HSAs to help shoulder their health costs than those enrolled in Medicare Advantage. As enrollment in HSAs has increased, the average household income for HSA account holders has dropped to $56,000 annually. With HSAs becoming more common at nearly every income demographic, we need to mold them to best fit the needs of Americans. Healthcare is not a one-size-fits-all situation; everyone has different needs. H.R.5138, "The Bipartisan HSA Improvement Act of 2018," offered by Congressmen Mike Kelly and Earl Blumenauer, will give consumers greater flexibility on how best to use their pre-tax medical funds. The provisions in H.R.5138, which include the PHIT Act, are common sense ways to make HSAs more useful in treating disease and promoting wellness, and ultimately bringing down the overall cost of healthcare. The committee is commended for working together to improve our healthcare model, and we strongly encourage you to pass bipartisan HSA reform to help consumers.

SFIA is happy to discuss the PHIT Act, HSA reform and the sedentary lifestyle problem with the committee.

Statement of Jane M. Orient, MD, Executive Director, Association of American Physicians and Surgeons, to: U. S. House Committee on Ways and Means, Subcommittee on Health, "Hearing on Lowering Costs and Expanding Access to Care through Consumer-Directed Plans," June 6, 2018

Chairman Roskam, Ranking Member Levin, and members of the Subcommittee,

We are asking you today to advance H. R. 365, the Primary Care Enhancement Act of 2017.

This 1-page bill has a simple goal: to allow patients to use their own Health Savings Accounts (HSAs) to pay for Direct Primary Care (DPC) service arrangements. These include all primary- care services, basic diagnostic tests, and commonly used prescription drugs at a package price. The bill clarifies that such arrangements are neither insurance nor health plans as defined in section 223(c) of the Internal Revenue Code and that they are payment for medical care under 213(d) of the code.

Passage of HR 365 is especially urgent since freeing HSAs to cooperate with DPC is a common sense policy that will augment the Administration's other coming policies to increase patient options, like the expansion of Association Health Plans and Short Term Limited Duration Insurance. The whole purpose of HSAs was to expand patients' freedom to choose how to spend their own money for medical care. More and more patients, including Medicare beneficiaries, are choosing DPC. They like the up-front, affordable price and the prompt access to a doctor they know and trust. Yet the current IRS interpretation of Internal Revenue Code will not allow patients with HSAs to use their own HSA funds for DPC agreements nor permit them to make tax deductible contributions to their HSA if they have a periodic DPC arrangement.

DPC is lowering costs for both patients and taxpayers. Prescription drugs accounted for $110 billion in Medicare spending in 2015, 17% of all

Medicare spending. With DPC dispensing, the cost of pharmaceuticals can be as much as 15 times lower than pharmacy prices. And $17 billion was spent on potentially avoidable hospital readmissions. DPC patients have fewer hospital admissions because of prompt, consistent, personalized care of chronic conditions, and fewer expensive emergency department visits because of 24-hour access to a physician who knows them.

It is improper for the IRS to be picking winners and losers in medical financing and care arrangements. It is counterproductive for a tax collection entity to discourage arrangements that save federal dollars while improving medical care. DPC also addresses the shortage of primary-care physicians by retaining physicians who would otherwise leave primary care practice or the profession altogether owing to "burn-out" from inability to serve their patients well under other practice models.

There is bipartisan support for this pro-patient bill, which advances all the goals of better access, lower cost, and higher quality. In addition, 1,125 physicians and patients from across the United States have signed a letter of support for this measure, sent earlier this month to Chairman Brady. The list of signers can be viewed at https://goo.gl/gm7wnZ.

Please expedite approval of H.R. 365 so that it can continue its path toward passage without further delay for the benefit of American patients. Thank you for your consideration.

Statement of Tracy Watts, Senior Partner Mercer, on Behalf of the American Benefits, Council and Mercer, before the Joint Economic Committee, Hearing on "The Potential for Health Care Savings Accounts to Engage Patients and Bend the Health Care Cost Curve," June 7, 2018

Chairman Paulsen, Ranking Member Heinrich, and Members of the Committee, thank you for this opportunity to meet with you to discuss the critical role health savings accounts are playing to help make health care more affordable.

My name is Tracy Watts, and I am a Senior Partner and US Healthcare Reform Leader at Mercer. I am testifying today on behalf of Mercer and the American Benefits Council, where I serve on their Policy Board of Directors. I have more than 30 years of experience in helping Fortune 500 companies design, finance and administer their health care programs and develop innovative plan designs to control costs and improve the quality of care.

Mercer is a business unit of Marsh & McLennan Companies (MMC), a US-based leading professional services firm with a global network of more than 65,000 experts in risk, strategy, and people. The businesses of MMC, including Mercer, Oliver Wyman, and Marsh & McLennan Agency, collaborate with our clients to navigate the increasingly complex healthcare marketplace to help individuals, families and employees stay healthy and productive, enable innovation, and lower costs.

Our company employs nearly 25,000 colleagues in the US, including more than more than 350 in your district, Chairman Paulsen.

The Council and Mercer appreciate the opportunity to participate in today's timely and critical hearing. The Council is a public policy organization representing principally Fortune 500 companies and other organizations that assist employers of all sizes in providing benefits to employees. Collectively, the Council's members either sponsor directly or provide services to retirement and health plans that cover more than 100 million Americans.

I would like to begin my testimony today by highlighting some important and very relevant findings from Mercer's most recent National Survey of Employer-Sponsored Health Care Plans. The survey, which includes responses from more than 2,500 employers, is the oldest, largest and most comprehensive survey of its kind withresults that are statistically valid and projectable for any size employer population in the US. I'll then describe some employer case studies and Mercer analyses that suggest employees enrolled in an HSA-eligible health plan get the care they need, have lower health care costs, and — most importantly — do a good job maintaining theirhealth.

The findings from our survey indicate that an increasing number of American workers and their families are enrolled in consumer-directed health plans ("CDHPs"), also known as account-based plans. Approximately 34% of covered employees working for large employers (those with 500 or more employees) were enrolled in a CDHP in 2017, which represents a rather astounding 325% increase since 2009.

In addition to demonstrating the increased reliance on CDHPs by the American worker, the results from our nationwide survey indicate that HSA-eligible plans save about 20% on plan costs when compared to PPO plans and are 6% less costly than PPO plans with deductibles over $1,000. I would note for the Committee that the success of HSA-eligible plans in reducing plan costs is one of the few strategies proven to help "bend the cost curve" and, in turn, help manage premium costs for employees.

When we look at what has been happening with PPO deductibles for small employers, those with less than 500 employees, the average deductible has crept up to almost $2,000 for an individual. For larger employers it is now around $1,000 for an individual. By contrast, the median deductible for an HSA-eligible plan is $1,750 for an individual but participants also have the benefit of an HSA. According to our survey, 77% of employers contribute to their employees' HSA accounts.

While this trend of employers shifting more responsibility for cost to employees has been underway for some time, the need to avoid the 40% "Cadillac Tax" accelerated the process. We've seen that the average PPO deductible has risen faster than the overall medical plan cost for the past few years, and employees have been moving out of PPOs and into CDHPs with even higher deductibles. While some employers may still have room to raise employee cost-share, there's a growing sense that we need additional strategies to slow cost growth that don't involve shifting more cost or responsibility to employees.

In addition to performing our nationwide survey, we also help clients evaluate the performance of their medical plans – not only from a cost perspective, but also from a care and coverage perspective.

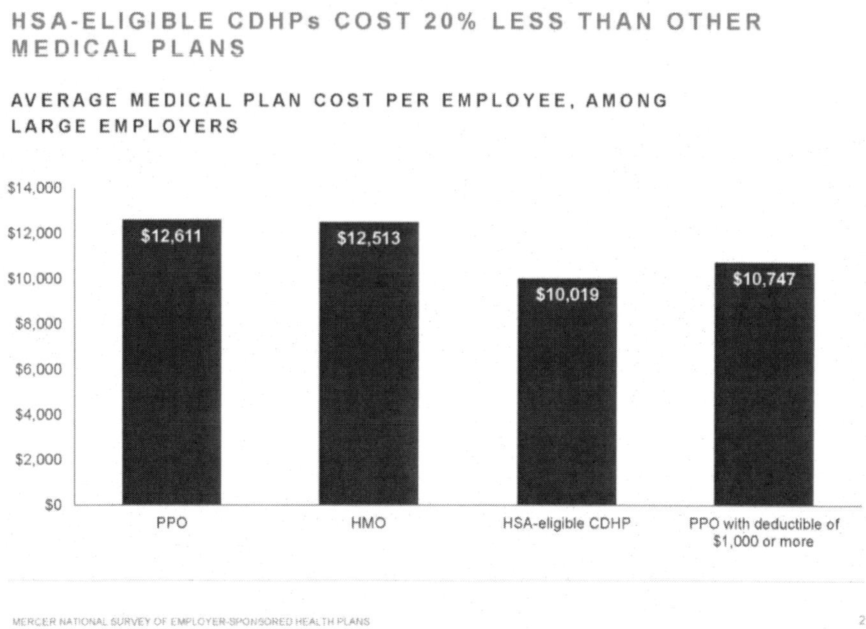

As part of my testimony today, I would like to share with the Committee an example of an analysis that we have done for some clients that best shows the actual positive effects of HSA-eligible plans on both cost and care.

In this case study, the employer had sponsored an HSA-eligible plan alongside a PPO plan for three years. We conducted a match analysis to compare and contrast the overall experience of approximately 26,000 individuals who were covered under either the employer's PPO or the HSA-eligible plan. To control for variances in health risks that could otherwise influence an individual's choice of plan option, we matched 13,000 individuals in the PPO with 13,000 enrollees in the HSA-eligible option who shared the same demographic and risk profiles at the start of the 3-year comparative period.

When we looked at how the participants in each of the plan options used their medical benefits, the data showed us that the utilization of health care was quite similar across the two groups. And while the HSA-eligible plan participants used slightly less care – with on average fewer emergency room visits and office visits – the HSA-eligible plan participants showed a slightly higher utilization of prescription medicines, which could actually mean they were more compliant with their prescribed therapies. As for preventive care, we also saw little difference between the two groups in their use of such care.

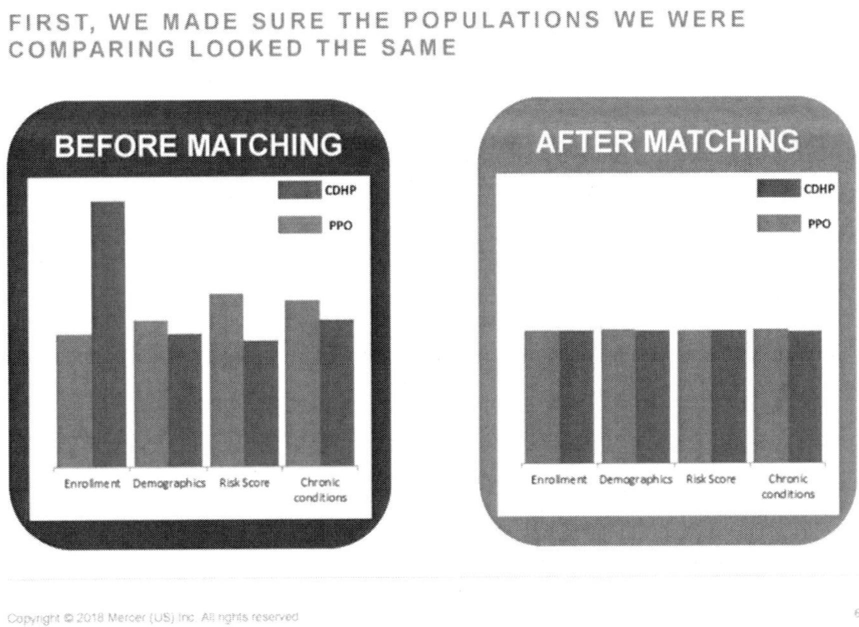

As mentioned, we sought to only compare individuals with similar demographic and risk characteristics across the two plans. One really interesting finding from this case study was that when we looked at the two groups over the three-year period, the HSA-eligible plan participants maintained their health status, while those in the PPO plan saw [on average] an 8% increase in identified health risks. This fact alone would seem to suggest that the HSA-eligible plan may have been more effective at helping participants mitigate the exacerbation of existing, or onset of new, medical conditions or health risks.

And, as for cost, the data was clear. The HSA-eligible plan ended up costing 15% less than the PPO plan over the 3-year period.

We performed similar analyses for several of our other employer clients and the results from these additional studies are very similar to those that I am sharing with you today.

Providing employees with the tools and resources to move toward consumer- directed health plans is a critical component. For employers that want to continue to provide employees with medical plan choices but would like to see greater enrollment in their high-deductible plans, enrollment results from our own Mercer Marketplace 365 benefit platform support the notion that more employees will choose to move into a high-deductible plan if they have the tools and resources to help them feel comfortable making that decision.

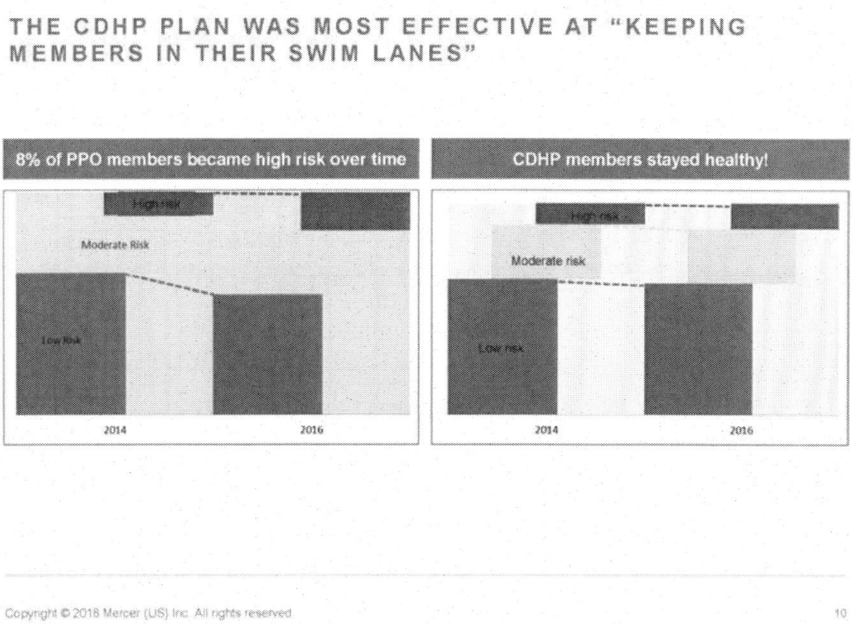

Finally, I want to note that in addition to the use of HSA-eligible plans, as well as other plans and coverage options, employers along with their consultants and advisors (such as Mercer) are developing innovative strategies to address some of the biggest cost drivers in the US healthcare system, including misplaced incentives, waste, uneven quality of care, and the lack of pricing and cost transparency.

Some strategies employers are pursing include implementing Centers of Excellence programs, creating on-site and near site health clinics so employees have easier access to care, implementing programs to better manage chronic conditions, and increased use of telemedicine. Unfortunately, many of these innovations are hamstrung by the HSA statute and regulations. For example, a patient with diabetes that is enrolled in an HSA-eligible HDHP must meet their entire deductible before the plan can cover an eye exam, foot exam, or diabetes medications.

Yet, the evidence is clear that patients with diabetes benefit from annual eye and foot exams and anti-diabetes medicines. Bipartisan bills have been introduced that change this. Additionally, employers can't waive cost-sharing for telemedicine, onsite clinics, Centers of Excellence, or second opinion services for employees that are enrolled in HSA-eligible HDHPs. These reforms would inject Value-Based Insurance Design into this very popular plan design.

Many of the innovations to date outlined in Mercer and the Council's report "Leading the Way: Employer Innovations in Health Coverage" have met with huge success and – if expanded and encouraged – have the potential to fundamentally improve health care for all Americans. Mercer and the Council have developed additional suggestions for enhancing HSAs and making other policy improvements to help build on these successes that we would be glad to share with you.

We thank you for holding this hearing today. We hope that the hearing serves to help build on these successes by highlighting how HSAs can, indeed, engage patients and bend the cost curve

Thank you again for the opportunity to share these findings with the Committee.

I'll be pleased to answer your questions.

Comments for the Record, United States House of Representatives, Committee on Ways and Means, Health Subcommittee, Lowering Costs and Expanding Access to Health Care through Consumer-Directed Health Plans, Wednesday, June 6, 2018, 11:00 AM

By Michael G. Bindner, Center for Fiscal Equity.

Chairman Roskam and Ranking Member Levin, thank you for the opportunity to submit these comments for the record to the House Ways and Means Health Subcommittee. They mirror our submission to the committee of May 17, 2016.

Proposals along the lines proposed have long been a part of our standard package of health care reforms. We have long advocated a conversion to catastrophic insurance with a medical savings account to pay for appointments and drugs, although we have always suggested a third element – a Medical Line of Credit to bridge the gap between the current MSA balance at the catastrophic deductible. The MLC would also pay for services, including acupuncture and reproductive health that may not be covered or coverable under catastrophic insurance.

Under our standard tax reform proposal, catastrophic policies would be purchased by all employers (and certain self-employed) as an offset to the Net Business Receipts Tax/Subtraction VAT. The Net Business Receipts Tax (NBRT) includes tax expenditures for family support, health care and the private delivery of governmental services. It will fund entitlement spending and replace income tax filing for most people (including people who file without paying), the corporate income tax, business tax filing through individual income taxes and the employer contribution to OASI, all payroll taxes for hospital insurance, disability insurance, unemployment insurance and survivors under age 60.

While this raises the tax rate, the lack of any tax subsidy would doom private insurance and deny most families medical care. Likewise, the

Health Savings Account would be provided by employers, but would be a deduction rather than a credit. Medical Lines of Credit would be funded entirely by employees with no tax advantage – as under our plan most employees would not pay any income taxes.

Personal experience with cardiac care (luckily a succession of false alarms) showed that, while this approach makes economic sense, it does not jibe with how doctors operate. There is no price schedule in the waiting or exam rooms to compare costs for proposed procedures or tests. Health care is not a normal good. While it responds to market pressures, some care cannot be limited by them.

I also came to the conclusion with the passage of health care reform – and the electoral rejection of the health care reform above which was not far from what Senator McCain proposed in his 2008 run (and which was not even mentioned as the Republican alternative in the Obamacare debate) – that Americans like their comprehensive insurance. Most importantly, while the Medical Line of Credit is essential for complete health care, its inclusion essentially short circuits any decision to shop for care.

If the McCain approach cannot pass, will the Affordable Care Act survive the test of time (it has certainly survived all attempts to repeal it)? Possibly. The key concept, that people in marginal jobs deserve the same tax subsidies that corporate employees get is sound. Those parts that fulfill that need, which originated in the Heritage Foundation (which even now clamors for repeal) are also worthy.

What is less defensible are the higher non-wage income taxes used to fund it, although no bill which just repeals these will survive a Budget Act point of order in the Senate (regardless of House Rules) nor would the political optics look good. Repeal would hurt too many Americans, so expansion of the tax (along with a rate cut) with some form of consumption or payroll tax– such as the one proposed by Senator Sanders in his single payer plan (or by Mrs. Clinton during her husband's health care reform effort). In our proposal, the consumption tax used would be the NBRT/Subtraction VAT.

The main danger to the Affordable Care Act is ease of entry and exit. If it is too easy to get in, then people will wait until they are sick to sign up.

After they are well, any plan will stop coverage if you stop sending in your monthly premium check. If enough people do that, rates go up and the cycle goes down. This eventually leads to a collapse in the system that can be fixed in one of two ways – give everyone cheap and mandatory health care or place health insurers into bankruptcy, like General Motors and Chrysler, and reorganize them into a single-payer system (without any congressional action). Had the leadership laid out this scenario, it might have stopped the Affordable Care Act – and insurance companies would have most assuredly stopped contributions to the GOP.

The low-cost system with catastrophic care would operate as above (and would hopefully include the Medical Lines of Credit). Single-payer care would be funded by the NBRT/Subtraction VAT. Such a tax is superior to the payroll tax proposed by Senator Sanders because it would hit profit. The upper-income payroll taxes for non- wage income would repealed and incorporated into the NBRT.

Under Single-Payer, we propose an additional option. Firms that provide direct health care, such as automobile manufacturers, would not pay for third party coverage at all. The cost of the coverage provided would be an offset to the NBRT.

We believe that our current insurance system adds no value to health care. Theoretically, insurance pools everyone's costs and divides them up with everyone paying a monthly share, regardless of the risk they pose.

The profit motive has given us differential premiums based on risk and age. Indeed, the age based premiums in the last attempted health reform were so unaffordable to older Americans in individual plans that the bill could not pass the Senate. Single payer plans, funded through the NBRT, would not have this feature and insurance companies doing claim processing for the government would be paid an adequate profit with little risk.

Short of that, an NBRT subsidized Public Option would allow sicker, poorer and older people to enroll for lower rates, allowing some measure of exclusion to private insurers and therefore lower costs. Of course, the profit motive will ultimately make the exclusion pool grow until private insurance would no longer be justified, leading-again to Single Payer if the race to cut customers leads to no one left in private insurance who is actually sick.

The NBRT can provide an incentive for cost savings if we allow employers to offer services privately to both employees and retirees in exchange for a substantial tax benefit, either by providing insurance or hiring health care workers directly and building their own facilities. Employers who fund catastrophic care or operate nursing care facilities would get an even higher benefit, with the proviso that any care so provided be superior to the care available through Medicaid. Making employers responsible for most costs and for all cost savings allows them to use some market power to get lower rates, but no so much that the free market is destroyed.

This proposal is probably the most promising way to arrest health care costs from their current upward spiral – as employers who would be financially responsible for this care through taxes would have a real incentive to limit spending in a way that individual taxpayers simply do not have the means or incentive to exercise.

While not all employers would participate, those who do would dramatically alter the market. In addition, a kind of beneficiary exchange could be established so that participating employers might trade credits for the funding of former employees who retired elsewhere, so that no one must pay unduly for the medical costs of workers who spent the majority of their careers in the service of other employers.

Thank you for the opportunity to address the committee. We are, of course, available for direct testimony or to answer questions by members and staff.

Michael Bindner
Center for Fiscal Equity

Health Subcommittee, Lowering Costs and Expanding Access to Health Care through Consumer-Directed Health Plans, Wednesday, June 6, 2018, 11:00 AM

All submissions must include a list of all clients, persons and/or organizations on whose behalf the witness appears:

This testimony is not submitted on behalf of any client, person or organization other than the Center itself, which is so far unfunded by any donations.

Statement for the Record, Committee on Ways and Means, Hearing on Lowering Costs and Expanding Access to Health Care through Consumer-Directed Health Plans, June 20, 2018

Chairman Roskam, Ranking Member Levin, and Members of the Subcommittee, the Council for Affordable Health Coverage (CAHC) appreciates the opportunity to submit a statement for the record on lowering costs and expanding access to health care through Consumer Directed Health Plans.

About CAHC

CAHC is a broad-based alliance with a singular focus: bringing down the cost of health care for all Americans. Our membership reflects a broad range of interests—organizations representing patient groups, consumers, small and large employers, insurers, and physician organizations. All told, we have more than 75 distinct member organizations representing tens of millions of people with an interest in more people covered in affordable private insurance arrangements, including consumer directed health plans paired with Health Savings Accounts (HSAs) and other account-based plans.

Health Costs Ascendant

CAHC is concerned health costs are too high and rising too fast. In fact, costs continue to rise faster than the economy and incomes.

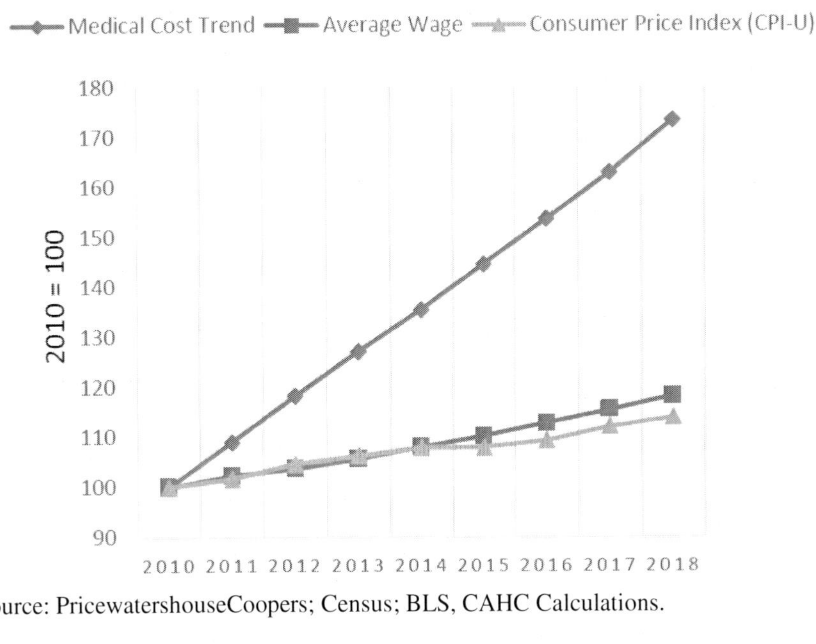

Source: PricewatershouseCoopers; Census; BLS, CAHC Calculations.

Last year, combined insurance and out-of-pocket spending in an average employer health plan for the typical family of four totaled $28,166 – up from "just" $9,435 in 2002.[63] Since 2010, the medical cost trend, which drives premiums and cost sharing, has increased by 73 percent,

[63] 2018 Milliman Medical Index available at http://www.milliman.com/mmi/.

about four times faster than wages. As a result, by 2030 the typical family will spend more than 50 percent of their income on health care.[64]

This is not sustainable.

Account Based Plans

HSAs, HRAs, FSAs and other account-based plans are lowering costs and proving more affordable alternatives to ACA or other plans for consumers and employers. HSAs allow consumers to put aside tax-free money to cushion the blow of rising health costs; they also create incentives for consumers to seek out the lowest cost, best quality care. To be maximally effective, therefore, consumers need transparency in health care.

First created in 2003, HSAs have gained widespread acceptance by employers and employees alike, but Congress has failed to upgrade the law to reflect market advances. These changes include flexible benefit designs, zero-dollar preventive care, wellness and telehealth strategies, and transparency tools to inform consumer decisions. In many ways, therefore, markets have outpaced the statutory construct of HSAs. CAHC recommends Congress enact reforms to modernize HSAs to make HSAs both more attractive and more viable.

CAHC has endorsed H.R. 5138, the Bipartisan HSA Improvement Act (Reps. Kelly and Blumenauer) and H.R. 4469, the Health Savings Act of 2016 (Rep. Paulsen), and encourages the Committee to move forward with the ideas contained in both bills. Specifically, CAHC supports the allowance of distributions for OTC drugs, preventive care clarification, direct primary care arrangements, workplace wellness programs and other changes to make HSAs work better for account holders and employers.

There are three additional challenges specific to HSAs that Congress should address, including:

---

64 "2015 Milliman Medical Index." Milliman, May 2015. http://www.milliman.com/uploadedFiles/insight/Periodicals/mmi/2015-MMI.pdf.

1) Providing flexibility for the insurance associated with HSAs by allowing plans to meet an actuarial value rather than the current strict statutory rules;
2) Clarifying the treatment of excepted benefits and allowing for coverage of telehealth services within the deductible; and
3) Ensuring better information on provider prices and quality to help drive better decisions and better tools.

Insurance Benefit Design Flexibility

Under current law, HSAs must be paired with acceptable insurance that meets certain statutory requirements, including a minimum deductible and a maximum out of pocket limit. Advances in insurance design, including value-based benefit design and modifications in cost sharing to meet certain actuarial values have become much more common since enactment of the HSA law.

CAHC supports providing more flexibility to employers and plans by allowing HSA affiliated insurance policies to meet an actuarial value of at least 70 percent of the statutory requirements. Plans should certify that their policies meet actuarial value based on the certification of private sector actuaries according to procedures determined by the Secretary of Treasury. This is based on the existing Part D model for certification of Actuarial Value for Part D plans and would allow insurers and employers to offer different benefit designs from a standard HSA-affiliated policy.

Excepted Benefits and Telehealth

Excepted benefit products are not major medical health insurance. "Excepted" benefits are defined in law (by Congress), they pre-date the ACA, and they are exempt from numerous provisions in the ACA, including its market reforms because these policies are not health insurance.

The 1996 HIPAA defined excepted benefits in statute and included "limited scope" dental and vision benefits, disability income, worker's compensation, long term care, and coverage for a specific disease or illness and hospital indemnity or fixed indemnity insurance. These benefit plans provide cash benefits and can replace lost income due to an illness or accident. Excepted benefits are not creditable coverage and are also not minimum essential coverage under the ACA, and individuals who have only excepted benefit coverage currently are still subject to the individual mandate penalty. Large employers that offer only excepted benefit coverage to their full-time employees must pay the employer mandate penalty if a worker accesses exchange subsidies.

CAHC supports a long-overdue technical correction to the 1996 HIPAA law that will conform the HSA "permitted insurance" text to the "excepted benefits" text that is used in ERISA, the Public Health Service Act, and other provisions of the Internal Revenue Code relating to "excepted benefits" insurance coverage. This "excepted benefits" technical correction will provide clarity to employers who are not always sure if a supplemental benefit they would like to provide is allowed to be offered alongside an HSA.

Finally, CAHC supports the expanded use of telehealth services because telehealth can improve access to care while lowering costs. Currently, telehealth services are covered medical expenses under HSA-affiliated group and individual health plans. HSA funds may be used to pay for these services and any associated cost sharing. We support allowing HSA-affiliated plans to cover telehealth within the deductible without impacting a person's eligibility for the HSA. The best way to achieve this goal is to treat telehealth as a separate issue from the excepted benefits issue and to clarify reimbursement for such services does not impacting HSA eligibility. We have attached language to this statement that achieves this goal.

Health Care Transparency

HSAs empower consumers to make choices about their health care by putting tax-free dollars in their hands. To stretch those dollars, they also need accurate information on plan, provider and drug costs. Last year combined insurance and out-of-pocket spending in an average employer health plan for the typical family of four totaled $28,166 – up from "just" $9,435 in 2002. The 2018 minimum annual deductible for self-only HDHP coverage is $1,350 (a $50 increase from 2017), while the family HDHP coverage is $2,700 (a $100 increase from 2017).[65] For those with Obamacare coverage, the average Silver plan deductible is $4,033. Consumers with higher deductibles tend to shop more, as depicted in the figure below and outlined in a 2017 Health Affairs study.[66]

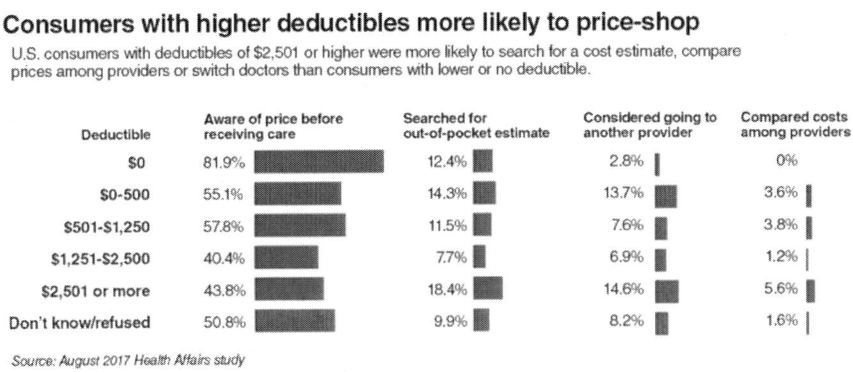

Unfortunately, consumers have more information on the price and quality of televisions than they do on health care providers. Most providers do not provide prices publicly, and if they do, the prices typically reflect "charges"—list prices—that often exceed actual amounts collected by several fold. In addition, prices within local markets can vary by as much as 700 percent. For example, MRIs are largely a commodity, but their price

---

[65] IRS https://www.irs.gov/pub/irs-drop/rp-17-37.pdf.

[66] Ateev Mehrotra, Katie M. Dean, Anna D. Sinaiko, and Neeraj Sood; Health Affairs, August 2017, "Americans Support Price Shopping For Health Care, But Few Actually Seek Out Price Information" accessed at https://www.healthaffairs.org/doi/pdf/10.1377/hlthaff.2016.1471.

varies greatly. If consumers knew price and quality of an imaging facility, they might choose a higher value provider. This creates competition and cost restraint.

CAHC's campaign on transparency has outlined a number of reforms we believe the Committee should pass as an add-on or side car to HSA modernization legislation. Below are some principles we encourage the Committee to consider:

- Provide consumers information on the price of the top 50 voluntary procedures. The price should be defined as an actual price (net of any price concessions) or as an average of all privately paid amounts, and ideally adjusted based on risk and complexity. 26 states have similar laws.
- In fact, some surgeons, surgery centers and hospitals are beginning to publish prices online. Knowledge of pricing is a wonderful start, but patients also need information on quality. Patients need tools to comparison-shop surgeons and facilities, so they get the most value.
- Uniformity in reporting is essential, so patients can become well-informed consumers. Reporting must be procedure-specific and include metrics such as number of cases performed, success rates and complication rates, all graded against national norms.
- Ultimately, we need to get to provider-specific, procedure-specific quality data, like number of cases performed, success rates and complication rates, so consumers can become well- informed shoppers.
- Private sector transparency tools are built off of data (price and quality) gleaned through claims, clinical and real-world data, which are often the byproduct of federal health programs, and, therefore, taxpayer investments. If released to the public, this data could be put to use to develop consumer tools, spot problems, and create solutions. HHS should be directed to increase the availability of health care data in standardized formats for developers, researchers, and consumers, for public good as by-

products of taxpayer investments in federal health programs. Congress should reform the QE program to expand access to provider data, including:

- Allowing insurers and employers to access the same raw data as providers;
- Reducing time for provider response to standardized reports;
- Expanding allowable uses of data and personal health information (Alternative Payment Models); and
- Allowing QEs to charge for data and value-add analytics.

Conclusion

While many Americans with significant health needs or lower incomes have greater access to coverage now, the reality is that for millions of others, health coverage is less affordable and more out of reach than when the ACA was enacted. Recent rate filings indicate this trend will continue and may worsen in the years to come. This fact should spur Congress to enact bipartisan reforms to expand consumer directed health plans to provide greater options that make health care more affordable and accessible for all Americans.

Telehealth Proposed amendment to 223(c)(2):

(E) A plan shall not fail to be treated as a high deductible health plan by reason of failing to have a deductible for telehealth services. For purposes of this section the term telehealth means the exchange of medical information from one site to another by means of electronic communications to improve a patient's clinical health status.

In: Health Insurance
Editor: Cory Oliver

ISBN: 978-1-53617-286-7

Chapter 3

INDIAN HEALTH SERVICE: FACILITIES REPORTED EXPANDING SERVICES FOLLOWING INCREASES IN HEALTH INSURANCE COVERAGE AND COLLECTIONS*

United States Government Accountability Office

ABBREVIATIONS

AI/AN	American Indian and Alaska Native
IHS	Indian Health Service
PPACA	Patient Protection and Affordable Care Act
PRC	Purchased/Referred Care.

* This is an edited, reformatted and augmented version of United States Government Accountability Office, Report to Congressional Requesters, Publication No. GAO-19-612, dated September 2019.

Why GAO Did This Study

IHS provides care to American Indians and Alaska Natives through a system of health care facilities. The Patient Protection and Affordable Care Act (PPACA) provided states with the option to expand their Medicaid programs, and created new coverage options beginning in 2014, including for American Indians and Alaska Natives. GAO was asked to review how PPACA has affected health care coverage and services for American Indians and Alaska Natives. In this chapter, GAO describes (1) trends in health insurance coverage and third-party collections at federally operated and tribally operated facilities from fiscal years 2013 through 2018, and (2) the effects of any changes in coverage and collections on these facilities.

To address these objectives, GAO analyzed IHS data on coverage, third-party collections, and PRC. GAO interviewed IHS officials from headquarters and all 12 area offices, as well as from 17 facilities selected to include a mix of federally operated and tribally operated hospitals and health centers in states that both had and had not expanded their Medicaid programs as of September 2018. GAO interviewed officials from 11 federally operated IHS facilities and 6 tribally operated facilities.

GAO provided a draft of this chapter to the Secretary of Health and Human Services for comment. The Department did not have any comments on the draft report.

What GAO Found

GAO's analysis of Indian Health Service (IHS) data shows that from fiscal years 2013 through 2018, the percent of patients at federally operated IHS hospitals and health centers that reported having health insurance coverage increased an average of 14 percentage points. While all federally operated IHS facilities reported coverage increases, the magnitude of these changes differed by facility, with those located in states that expanded access to Medicaid experiencing the largest increases. Federally operated

IHS facilities' third-party collections—that is, payments for enrollees' medical care from public programs such as Medicaid and Medicare, or from private insurers—totaled $1.07 billion in fiscal year 2018, increasing 51 percent from fiscal year 2013. Although exact figures were not available, tribally operated facilities, which include hospitals and health centers not run by IHS, also experienced increases in coverage and collections over this period, according to officials from selected facilities and national tribal organizations.

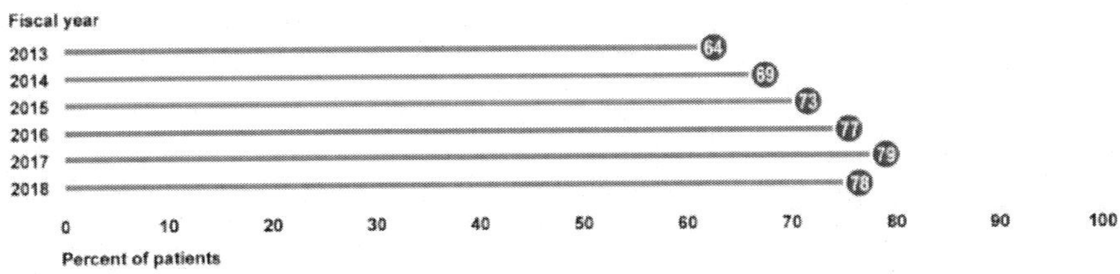

Source: GAO analysis of Indian Health Service (IHS) data. | GAO-19-612.

Note: Data represent patients' self-reported coverage information at each of the 73 federally operated IHS hospitals and health centers, averaged across the facilities, and do not reflect coverage through the Department of Veterans Affairs.

Average Percent of Patients at Federally Operated IHS Facilities Reporting Health Insurance Coverage, Fiscal Years 2013 through 2018.

Increases in health insurance coverage and third-party collections helped federally operated and tribally operated facilities continue their operations and expand the services offered, according to officials from 17 selected facilities. These officials told GAO that their facilities have been increasingly relying on third-party collections to pay for ongoing operations including staff payroll and facility maintenance. Officials at most facilities with increases in third-party collections also stated that they expanded their onsite services, including increasing the volume or scope of services offered by, for example, adding new providers or purchasing medical equipment. Increased coverage and collections also allowed for an expansion in the complexity of services provided offsite through the Purchased/Referred Care (PRC) program, which enables patients to obtain needed care from private providers if the patients meet certain requirements and funding is available. According to IHS and facility officials, increases in coverage have allowed some patients to access care offsite using their coverage, and an expansion of onsite services has reduced the need for some patients to access PRC. Officials GAO interviewed from federally operated and tribally operated facilities stated that facilities' expansion of onsite and offsite services has led to enhancements in patients' access to care in some instances.

September 3, 2019

The Honorable Frank Pallone, Jr.
Chair
Committee on Energy and Commerce
House of Representatives

The Honorable Raul Ruiz, MD
House of Representatives

The Indian Health Service (IHS) is responsible for providing health care for over two million American Indians and Alaska Natives (AI/AN) who are members or descendants of federally recognized tribes.[1] According to IHS, its mission is to raise the physical, mental, social, and spiritual health of AI/AN to the highest level. IHS provides health care services to AI/AN either directly through a system of federally operated IHS facilities or indirectly through facilities that are operated by tribes or others.[2] As of February 2019, IHS, tribes, and tribal organizations operated

---

[1] Federally recognized tribes have a government-to-government relationship with the United States and are eligible to receive certain protections, services, and benefits by virtue of their status as Indian tribes. The Secretary of the Interior publishes annually in the Federal Register a list of all tribal entities that the Secretary recognizes as Indian tribes. As of February 2, 2019, there were 573 federally recognized tribes. See 84 Fed. Reg. 1200 (Feb. 1, 2019).

[2] Under the Indian Self-Determination and Education Assistance Act, as amended, federally recognized Indian tribes can enter into self-determination contracts or self-governance compacts with the Director of IHS to take over the administration of IHS programs previously administered by IHS on their behalf. See generally 25 U.S.C. §§ 5301-5423. In fiscal year 2019, IHS allocated over 60 percent of its appropriations to tribes and tribal

46 hospitals and 353 health centers as well as a range of other types of health facilities—of which 24 hospitals and 50 health centers were federally operated IHS facilities. With almost 5 million outpatient visits in fiscal year 2017, federally operated IHS facilities provide mostly primary and emergency care, as well as some other services, and are located in ten of IHS's twelve geographic areas.[3] In certain circumstances when needed health care services are not available at federally operated or tribally operated facilities, care may be obtained from private providers and paid for through IHS's Purchased/Referred Care (PRC) program.

AI/AN have experienced long-standing problems accessing needed health care services and have historically had poorer health than the U.S. general population, as evidenced by a shorter average life span and higher incidence of certain medical conditions—many of which can be mitigated through access to effective preventive primary care services. In prior reports we have noted that IHS has not been able to pay for all eligible health care services, leading to an unmet need for health care among AI/AN.[4] In February 2017, GAO added federal management of programs that serve Indian tribes and their members to our High Risk List because inadequate oversight hindered IHS's ability to ensure that Indian communities have timely access to quality health care, among other reasons.[5]

Like most federal agencies, IHS receives funding through annual appropriations, which it uses to fund federally operated and tribally

---

organizations to operate part or all of their own health care programs through self-determination contracts and self-governance compacts. Under the Indian Health Care Improvement Act, IHS also awards contracts and grants to non-profit urban Indian organizations that provide health care and referral services to urban Indians; however, this chapter does not include a review of such facilities.

[3] The twelve IHS areas are Alaska, Albuquerque, Bemidji, Billings, California, Great Plains, Nashville, Navajo, Oklahoma City, Phoenix, Portland, and Tucson.

[4] GAO, *Indian Health Service: Health Care Services Are Not Always Available to Native Americans*, GAO-05-789 (Washington, D.C.: Aug. 31, 2005), and *Increased Oversight Needed to Ensure Accuracy of Data Used for Estimating Contract Health Service Need*, GAO-11-767 (Washington, D.C.: Sept. 23, 2011).

[5] The recommendations GAO identified in this high-risk area are neither reflective of the performance of programs administered by tribes nor directed at any tribally operated programs and activities. See GAO, *High-Risk Series: Progress on Many High-Risk Areas, While Substantial Efforts Needed on Others,* GAO-17-317 (Washington, D.C.: Feb. 15, 2017).

operated facilities throughout the country. These facilities may also bill public programs such as Medicaid (the federal-state health insurance program for certain low-income individuals), Medicare (the federal health insurance program for persons aged 65 and over, and certain others), and the Department of Veterans Affairs (which provides health care services for veterans), as well as private insurance, for care provided to patients.[6] Federally operated and tribally operated facilities are allowed to retain collections from these payers—referred to as third-party collections—without an offset to any other appropriations made to IHS.[7] Unlike funds made available through annual appropriations acts, which generally must be obligated during the fiscal year for which they were appropriated, third-party collections are available to facilities until expended.

Beginning in 2014, the Patient Protection and Affordable Care Act (PPACA) provided opportunities to expand coverage of AI/AN through Medicaid and private health insurance.[8] PPACA also provided that IHS is the payer of last resort for all health services provided at federally operated and tribally operated facilities—meaning that enrollees' health insurance coverage should pay for care, to the extent of its liability, before IHS. Increased AI/AN enrollment in health insurance such as Medicaid may increase revenue for federally operated and tribally operated facilities, even if the patient population remains constant, if those with coverage seek care at such facilities. Health insurance may also provide AI/AN with options to obtain care outside of federally operated or tribally operated facilities, including more comprehensive health services, if such options exist in their community.

In 2013, we reported that most AI/AN were potentially eligible for expanded coverage created by PPACA, but action was needed to increase

---

[6] 25 U.S.C. §§ 1621e(a), 1621f(a).

[7] See 25 U.S.C. § 1621(b).

[8] Specifically, PPACA provided states with the option to expand Medicaid eligibility to certain adults with incomes below a threshold; required the establishment of health insurance exchanges; and provided certain AI/AN with cost sharing exemptions for private health insurance plans purchased on the health insurance exchanges. Pub. L. No. 111- 148, 124 Stat. 119 (2010), as amended by the Health Care and Education Reconciliation Act of 2010, Pub. L. No. 111-152, 124 Stat. 1029. For purposes of this chapter, references to PPACA include the amendments made by the Health Care and Education Reconciliation Act of 2010.

enrollment.[9] You asked us to review how PPACA has affected AI/AN access to health care. In this chapter we describe, for fiscal years 2013 through 2018,

1. trends in health insurance coverage among AI/AN populations served by federally operated and tribally operated facilities as well as trends in third-party collections at these facilities, and
2. the effects of any changes in health insurance coverage and third-party collections on federally operated and tribally operated facilities.

To describe trends in health insurance coverage among AI/AN populations served by federally operated and tribally operated facilities, we analyzed IHS data representing the self-reported health insurance status of patients seeking care at all 73 federally operated IHS hospitals and health centers that were in operation from fiscal years 2013 through 2018.[10] We also analyzed IHS data on the amount and source of third-party collections at all IHS facilities—including hospitals, health centers, health clinics or other types of facilities—that were federally operated throughout this period.[11] We assessed the reliability of these data by reviewing related documentation, interviewing IHS officials, and examining the data for missing values and outliers.

[9] GAO, *Indian Health Service: Most American Indians and Alaska Natives Potentially Eligible for Expanded Health Coverage, but Action Needed to Increase Enrollment,* GAO-13-553 (Washington, D.C.: Sept. 5, 2013).

[10] While there were 74 federally operated IHS hospitals and health centers in operation as of fiscal year 2018, one of these did not routinely provide billable services during this time period, according to IHS officials, and is not included in our analysis. The 73 federally operated IHS hospitals and health centers included 47 facilities located in 11 states that had expanded Medicaid as of September 2018, and 26 located in 8 states that had not.

[11] Our analysis of IHS's third-party collections at federally operated facilities reflects collections at all such facilities in operation from fiscal years 2013 through 2018, including the 73 federally operated hospitals and health clinics included in our analysis of changes in coverage. The collections data were provided to us in an aggregated format that included 40 federally operated service units (which may contain one or more facilities) as well as 45 individual facilities such as hospitals, health centers, and smaller health clinics. Service units may cover a number of small reservations, or, conversely, some large reservations may be covered by several service units.

On the basis of these steps, we concluded that the data were sufficiently reliable for the purposes of our reporting objective. Similar aggregate data on trends in health insurance coverage and collections at tribally operated facilities are not available because these facilities are not required to report coverage and collections data to IHS. For information and context on trends in coverage and collection at federally operated and tribally operated facilities, we interviewed officials from IHS headquarters and all 12 area offices, as well as those from 17 facilities, which we selected to include a mix of federally operated and tribally operated facilities, including hospitals and health centers ranging in size and location and those operating in states that had expanded their Medicaid programs as of September 2018 as well as those that had not.[12] In total, we interviewed officials from 11 federally operated facilities and 6 tribally operated facilities across 7 states, with 14 facilities located in states that expanded Medicaid, and 3 located in states that had not. Our findings from these interviews cannot be generalized to all federally operated or tribally operated facilities. For context, we also interviewed officials from the National Indian Health Board, five area Indian health boards which we selected to include a mix of areas with predominantly tribal facilities as well as those with federally operated and tribally operated facilities, as well as officials from the National Congress of American Indians and the Tribal Self-Governance Advisory Committee.[13]

---

[12] We interviewed officials from the following 11 federally operated IHS facilities: Blackfeet Community Hospital, Cass Lake Hospital, Chemawa Indian Health Center, Claremore Indian Hospital, Lawton Indian Hospital, Not-Tsoo Gah-nee Indian Health Center, Phoenix Indian Medical Center, Red Lake Hospital, White Earth Health Center, Whiteriver Indian Hospital, and Yakama Indian Health Center. We also interviewed officials from the following six tribally operated facilities: Cow Creek Health and Wellness Center, Inchelium Community Health Center, Jamestown Family Health Clinic, San Carlos Apache Healthcare Corporation, San Poil Valley Community Health Center, and Yellowhawk Tribal Health Center.

[13] The National Indian Health Board is a nonprofit organization that represents tribal governments—both those that operate their own health care delivery systems through contracting and compacting, and those receiving health care directly from the Indian Health Service (IHS). Among other things, it provides policy analysis and advocacy on AI/AN health issues. Area Indian health boards are organizations that advocate for the health needs of tribes in geographic regions that largely align with those supported by IHS's area offices. We interviewed officials from the Alaska Native Health Board, California Rural Indian Health Board, Inter Tribal Council of Arizona, Inc., Northwest Portland Area Indian Health

To describe the effects of any changes in health insurance coverage and third-party collections on federally operated and tribally operated facilities from fiscal years 2013 through 2018, we interviewed IHS officials, including those at headquarters and all 12 area offices, as well as officials from the 17 selected facilities. We also interviewed officials from the five selected area Indian health boards, and the three selected national tribal organizations. We asked these officials to identify the effects of changes in coverage and collections. Our findings from these interviews cannot be generalized to all federally operated or tribally operated facilities. We also analyzed IHS data on the scope of care provided through IHS's PRC program from fiscal year 2015—the first year data were available— through fiscal year 2018.[14] This IHS data reflect care provided through IHS-administered PRC programs, which represented 39 percent of total PRC appropriations in fiscal year 2018; similar data on the scope of care provided through tribally-administered PRC programs, which account for the remaining portion of PRC appropriations, were not available because such data are not required to be reported to IHS. We assessed the reliability of these data by interviewing IHS officials and examining the data for missing values and outliers. On the basis of these steps, we concluded that the data were sufficiently reliable for the purposes of our reporting objective.

We conducted this performance audit from July 2018 through September 2019 in accordance with generally accepted government auditing standards. Those standards require that we plan and perform the audit to obtain sufficient, appropriate evidence to provide a reasonable basis for our findings and conclusions based on our audit objectives. We believe that the evidence obtained provides a reasonable basis for our findings and conclusions based on our audit objectives.

Board, and United South and Eastern Tribes, Inc. The National Congress of American Indians is a nonprofit organization that promotes the economic development and health and welfare in AI/AN communities, among other things. The Tribal Self-Governance Advisory Committee provides information, education, advocacy and policy guidance for implementation of self-governance within IHS.

[14] Fiscal year 2015 represents the first year that IHS collected national data on the scope of care provided through IHS-administered PRC programs.

BACKGROUND

Indian Health Service

IHS was established within the Public Health Service in 1955 in order to meet federal treaty obligations to provide health services to members of federally recognized AI/AN tribes primarily in rural areas on or near reservations. IHS oversees its provision of health care services through a decentralized system of 12 area offices, which are led by area directors and located in 12 geographic areas.[15] IHS's headquarters office is responsible for setting national health care policy, ensuring the delivery of quality comprehensive health services, and advocating for the health needs and concerns of AI/AN people. The area offices are responsible for monitoring federally operated IHS facilities' operations and finances, and providing guidance and technical assistance.

Table 1. Indian Health Service Federally Operated and Tribally Operated Facilities, as of February 2019

Facility type	Federal	Tribal	Total
Hospital	24	22	46
Health centers	50	303	353
Other facilities[a]	35	308	343
Total	109	633	742

Source: Indian Health Service. | GAO-19-612. [a]Other facilities include health stations and school health clinics, which provide primary care services and are open less than 40 hours a week, as well as Alaska village clinics, dental clinics, and substance abuse treatment facilities.

IHS's 12 area offices oversee 168 service units which provide care at the local level through a total of 742 federally operated and tribally operated hospitals, health centers, and other health facilities. The types of services offered by these facilities vary, but most commonly include

[15] As of fiscal year 2018, nine of these twelve IHS areas had two or more federally operated IHS facilities—Albuquerque, Bemidji, Billings, Great Plains, Nashville, Navajo, Oklahoma City, Phoenix, and Portland. In fiscal year 2018, the California area had one federally operated IHS facility and the Alaska and Tucson areas had no federally operated IHS facilities.

primary care and emergency care, as well as some ancillary and specialty services.[16] Table 1 displays the number of federally operated and tribally operated facilities as of February 2019.

PRC Program

If federally operated or tribally operated facilities are unable to provide needed care, they may contract for health services from private providers through the PRC program. Patients must meet certain eligibility and administrative requirements in order to qualify for this care—including having exhausted all other health care resources available to them and living on a federally recognized Indian reservation or within a designated PRC delivery area.[17]

The PRC program is funded through the annual appropriations process and administered at the local level by individual PRC programs that are often affiliated with local facilities. Individual PRC programs may be federally or tribally administered, and as of fiscal year 2018, IHS administered 39 percent of PRC appropriations, and tribes administered the remaining 61 percent.

PRC funding is limited and has traditionally been reserved for the most critical cases. IHS has established five medical priority levels. Funds permitting, federally administered PRC programs first pay for all of the

[16] For example, federally operated IHS hospitals range in size from 4 to 133 beds and are open 24 hours a day for urgent care needs. Federally operated IHS health centers offer a range of care, including primary care services and some ancillary services, such as pharmacy, laboratory, and X-ray, and are open for at least 40 hours a week. Other federally operated IHS facilities include health stations and school health clinics, which provide primary care services and are open less than 40 hours per week.

[17] PRC delivery areas typically encompass reservation and trust lands—areas located on or off a reservation, for which the United States holds title in trust for the benefit of a tribe or individual Indian—and bordering counties. AI/AN living outside of these areas, which may include many urban Indians, are therefore unlikely to be eligible for PRC.

highest priority services, and then all or some of the lower priority services.[18] IHS's five PRC medical priority levels are

1. Emergent and acutely urgent care services, which include treatment for threats to life, limb, or senses;
2. Preventive care services, which include prenatal care and mammograms;
3. Primary and secondary care services, which include scheduled ambulatory services for nonemergent conditions, and specialty consultations;
4. Chronic tertiary and extended care services, which include rehabilitation care, skilled nursing facility care, and organ transplants; and
5. Excluded services, which include cosmetic and experimental procedures.

PPACA Health Coverage Expansion Provisions for AI/AN

Beginning in 2014, PPACA allowed states to expand Medicaid eligibility to non-elderly, non-pregnant adults who are not eligible for Medicare and whose income does not exceed 133 percent of the federal poverty level.[19] As of September 2018, there were 32 "expansion states"—those states including the District of Columbia that chose to expand

---

[18] Federally administered PRC programs must use these levels to prioritize funding for medical care, whereas tribally administered PRC programs may establish their own mechanisms for funding care.

[19] PPACA provides a 5 percent disregard when calculating income for determining Medicaid eligibility, which effectively increases income eligibility from 133 percent to 138 percent of the federal poverty level. See Pub. L. No. 111-148, §§ 2001(a)(1), 2002, 124 Stat. 119, 271, 279 (2010); Pub. L. No. 111-152, § 1004(e), 124 Stat. 1029, 1034 (2010) (codified at 42 U.S.C. § 1396a(a)(10)(A)(i)(VIII) and 42 U.S.C. § 1396a(e)(14)(B)(I)). The federal poverty level is based on household income and family size, using the U.S. Census Bureau's poverty thresholds. For 2018, 138 percent of the federal poverty level for those residing in the contiguous United States or the District of Columbia was $16,753 for an individual and $34,638 for a family of four; amounts are higher for those living in Alaska and Hawaii. PPACA also permitted an early expansion option, whereby states could expand eligibility for this population, or a subset of this population, starting on April 1, 2010.

Medicaid eligibility to this additional adult population—and 19 "non-expansion states"—those that had not expanded Medicaid eligibility.[20]

PPACA also required the establishment of health insurance exchanges in 2014—marketplaces where individuals may compare and select among health insurance plans offered by participating private insurers. PPACA included a number of provisions that reduced these plans' costs—including premiums and cost-sharing, such as deductibles and copayments—for eligible enrollees, including certain AI/AN.[21]

HEALTH INSURANCE COVERAGE AND THIRD-PARTY COLLECTIONS AT FEDERALLY OPERATED IHS FACILITIES INCREASED FROM 2013 TO 2018; TRIBAL FACILITY OFFICIALS ALSO REPORTED INCREASES

IHS Data Show Increase in Percent of Patients with Health Insurance Coverage at Federally Operated IHS Facilities from 2013 through 2018

Our analysis of IHS data shows that from fiscal year 2013 through fiscal year 2018, the percent of patients at 73 federally operated IHS

[20] Specifically, the 31 states that expanded their Medicaid programs as of September 2018 were Alaska, Arizona, Arkansas, California, Colorado, Connecticut, Delaware, Hawaii, Illinois, Indiana, Iowa, Kentucky, Louisiana, Maryland, Massachusetts, Michigan, Minnesota, Montana, Nevada, New Hampshire, New Jersey, New Mexico, New York, North Dakota, Ohio, Oregon, Pennsylvania, Rhode Island, Vermont, Washington, and West Virginia. States that had not expanded their Medicaid programs as of September 2018 were Alabama, Florida, Georgia, Idaho, Kansas, Maine, Mississippi, Missouri, Nebraska, North Carolina, Oklahoma, South Carolina, South Dakota, Tennessee, Texas, Utah, Virginia, Wisconsin, and Wyoming.

[21] Specifically, PPACA offers a premium tax credit for enrollees purchasing coverage on the exchange that have household incomes between 100 and 400 percent of the federal poverty level. PPACA also offers cost-sharing reductions for enrollees who qualify for premium tax credits, have household incomes between 100 and 250 percent of the federal poverty level, and enroll in a silver tier plan. In addition, AI/AN who obtain insurance through an exchange are eligible for cost-sharing exemptions if they are members of federally recognized tribes and have a household income of not more than 300 percent of the federal poverty level. Pub. L. No. 111-148, § 1402(d)(1), 124 Stat. 119, 222 (2010) (codified at 42 U.S.C. § 18071(d)(1)).

hospitals and health centers who reported having health insurance coverage increased an average of 14 percentage points, from 64 percent in fiscal year 2013 to 78 percent in fiscal year 2018.[22] The majority of coverage gains occurred in fiscal years 2014 through 2016 (see Figure 1).[23]

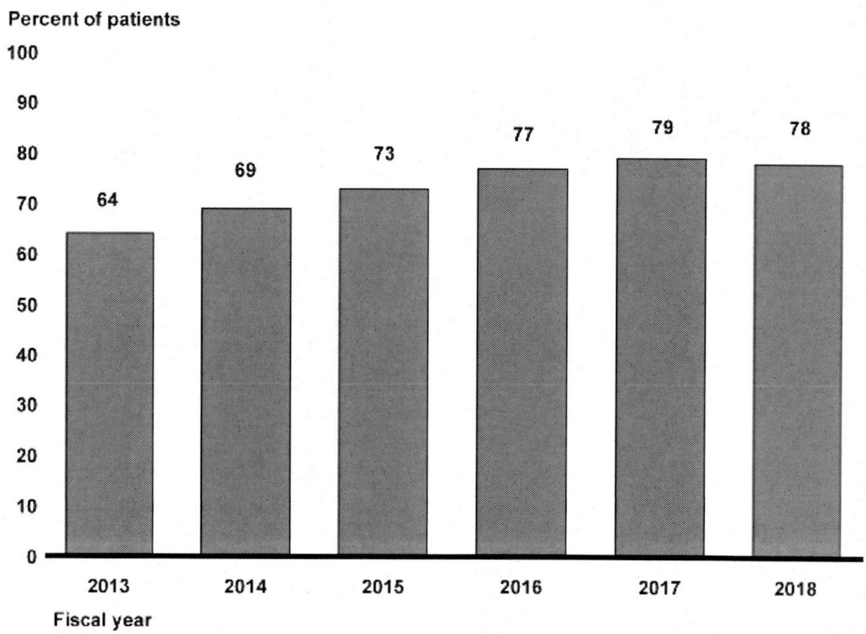

Source: GAO analysis of Indian Health Service (IHS) data. | GAO-19-612.

Note: Data represent patients' self-reported coverage information at each of the 73 federally operated IHS hospitals and health centers, averaged across the facilities, and do not reflect coverage through the Department of Veterans Affairs.

Figure 1. Average Percent of Patients at Federally Operated IHS Facilities Reporting Health Insurance Coverage, Fiscal Year 2013 through Fiscal Year 2018.

---

[22] Data represent patients' self-reported coverage information collected during patient registration. Percentages from each of the federally operated IHS hospitals and health centers were averaged across the 73 facilities. Results do not reflect coverage through the Department of Veterans Affairs.

[23] Trends in coverage at federally operated IHS facilities mirror those seen in the general AI/AN population. For more information about trends in health insurance coverage of the AI/AN population, see Appendix I.

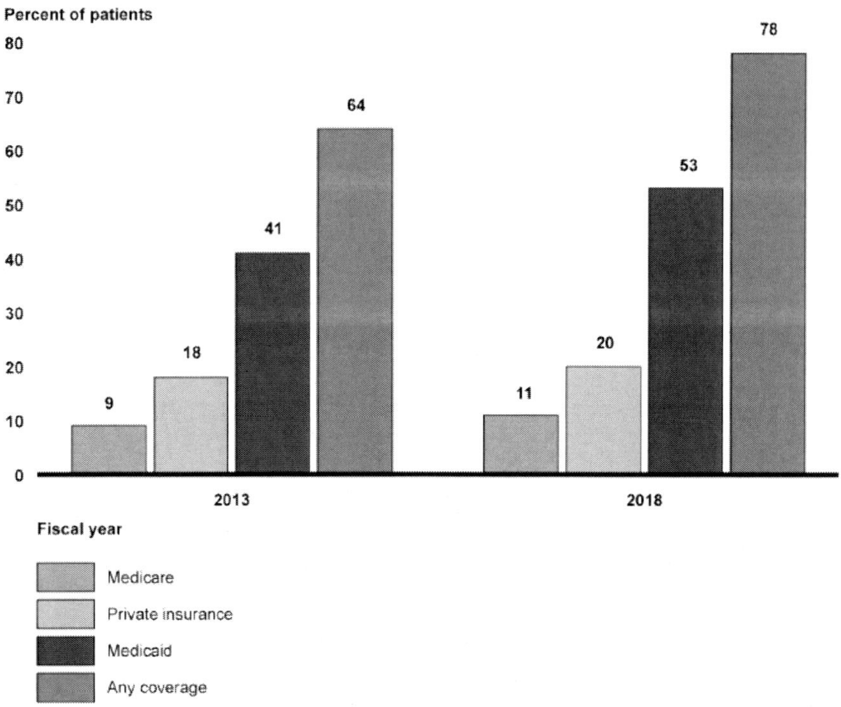

Source: GAO analysis of Indian Health Service (IHS) data. | GAO-19-612.

Notes: Data represent patients' self-reported coverage information at each of the 73 federally operated IHS hospitals and health centers, averaged across the facilities, and do not reflect coverage through the Department of Veterans Affairs. Coverage type categories are not mutually exclusive and therefore do not sum to 100 percent. For example, a patient may have both Medicare and private insurance coverage. Any coverage includes patients that report having coverage through Medicaid, private insurance, Medicare, or any combination of those coverage types.

Figure 2 Average Percent of Patients Reporting Health Insurance Coverage at Federally Operated IHS Facilities, by Year and Coverage Type, Fiscal Year 2013 and Fiscal Year 2018.

Patients at federally operated IHS facilities reported obtaining health insurance coverage from several sources. The largest increase in coverage occurred among those reporting Medicaid coverage. On average, 41 percent of IHS patients in fiscal year 2013 reported they had coverage through Medicaid at some point during the year; this number increased to

53 percent in fiscal year 2018. In comparison, the percent of patients at each facility who reported having Medicare and the percent who reported having private insurance at some point during the year each increased an average of two percentage points from fiscal years 2013 to 2018.[24] (See Figure 2).

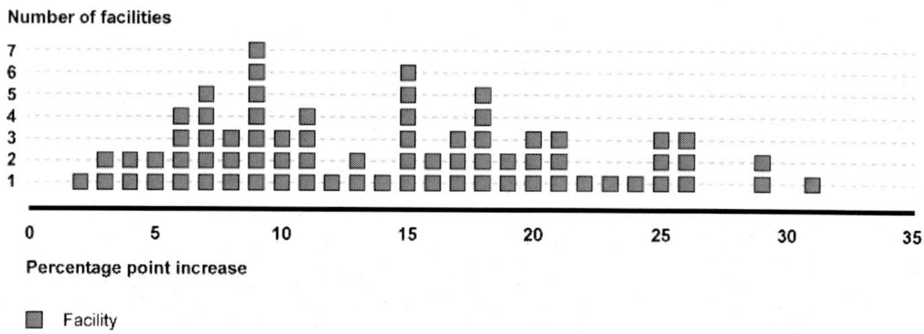

Source: GAO analysis of Indian Health Service (IHS) data. | GAO-19-612.

Note: Data represent patients' self-reported coverage information from 73 federally operated IHS hospitals and health centers, and do not reflect coverage through the Department of Veterans Affairs.

Figure 3. Distribution of Percentage Point Increase in Patient-Reported Health Insurance Coverage at Federally Operated IHS Facilities, Fiscal Years 2013 through 2018.

While the average percent of patients reporting health care coverage increased across all federally operated IHS facilities, our analysis of IHS data showed substantial variation in the magnitude of these increases. Specifically, from fiscal year 2013 through fiscal year 2018, increases at each of the 73 facilities ranged from a low of 2 to a high of 31 percentage points. Forty-four federally operated IHS facilities experienced an increase in the percent of patients with coverage over this time period of more than 10 percentage points (see Figure 3).

Our analysis of IHS data shows that federally operated IHS facilities in states that expanded Medicaid had larger increases in health insurance coverage compared with such facilities in states that had not expanded Medicaid. Specifically, federally operated IHS facilities in Medicaid

[24] Coverage type categories are not mutually exclusive and therefore do not sum to 100 percent.

expansion states experienced an average 17 percentage point increase in patients reporting any form of health coverage, compared with an average 8 percentage point increase at federally operated IHS facilities in states that did not expand Medicaid.[25] However, these increases in coverage were not spread evenly among the facilities. (See Figure 4).

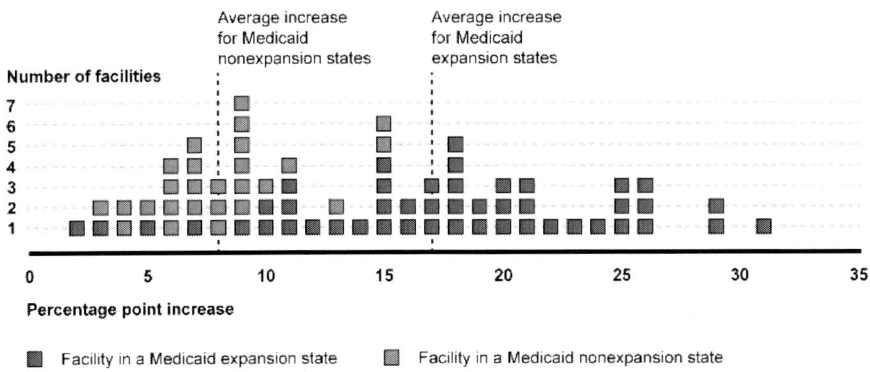

Source: GAO analysis of Indian Health Service (IHS) data. | GAO-19-612.

Note: Data represent patients' self-reported coverage information from 73 federally operated IHS hospitals and health centers, and do not reflect coverage through the Department of Veterans Affairs.

Figure 4. Distribution of Percentage Point Increase in Patient-Reported Health Insurance Coverage at Federally Operated IHS Facilities, by State Medicaid Expansion Status, Fiscal Years 2013 through 2018.

IHS officials we interviewed also reported that a variety of factors in addition to Medicaid expansion likely affected the number of patients at federally operated IHS facilities who reported having health insurance coverage. Specifically, officials we interviewed at all of the 11 selected federally operated IHS facilities cited efforts at their facilities that helped increase coverage, such as increasing the number of onsite patient benefits coordinators to help enroll patients in all forms of health coverage and enhancing efforts to ensure that all patients were screened for coverage. For example, one federally operated IHS facility reported renovating its

[25] Data reflect the experience of 47 federally operated IHS facilities located across 11 states that expanded Medicaid and 26 federally operated IHS facilities located across 8 states that did not expand Medicaid.

office to, among other things, move the patient benefits coordinator near the waiting room, which allowed patients to be immediately screened after walking in for an appointment. Officials we interviewed at nearly all of the selected federally operated IHS facilities also noted that their outreach and education efforts about the importance of health insurance coverage may have helped to increase enrollment. Officials we interviewed at all of the selected federally operated IHS facilities said they were engaged in such activities which included broadcasting public service announcements, posting newspaper advertisements, and promoting insurance during community events. Officials from most of the 12 IHS area offices also reported collaborating with tribes to conduct outreach and education to enhance enrollment.

Officials at many IHS area offices also noted that external factors may have also played a role in increasing coverage levels, such as improvements in the local economy, which officials said led to increases in the number of patients with private health insurance. Additionally, entities outside of IHS also implemented initiatives to increase coverage for patients at federally operated IHS facilities. For example, IHS officials stated that some patients obtained health insurance through the health insurance exchanges, and in some cases, the tribe paid all premiums, coinsurance, and deductibles for these plans. In addition, a number of area Indian health boards worked together to develop a train-the-trainer program to disseminate information and resources to encourage enrollment and share information on the benefits of having health coverage.

Total Third-Party Collections at Federally Operated IHS Facilities Increased 51 Percent from Fiscal Years 2013 through 2018

Third-party collections across all federally operated IHS facilities increased 51 percent from fiscal year 2013 through fiscal year 2018, according to our analysis of IHS data. Specifically, total third-party collections increased from $708 million in fiscal year 2013 to about $1.07

billion in fiscal year 2018 while the number of patients seeking care remained constant.[26] Medicaid collections accounted for 65 percent of the total $360 million increase, though collections from Medicare, private insurance, and Veterans Affairs also increased during this period. For example, Medicaid collections grew 47 percent, from $496 million in fiscal year 2013 to $729 million in fiscal year 2018. (See Figure 5).

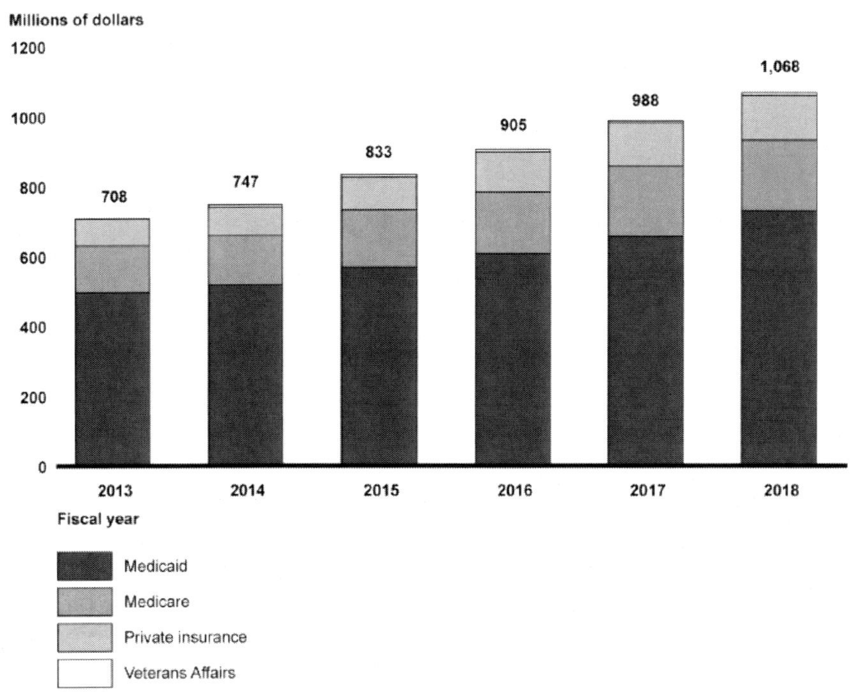

Source: GAO analysis of Indian Health Service (IHS) data. | GAO-19-612.
Note: Third-party collections are presented in nominal dollars.

Figure 5. Total Collections for Federally Operated IHS Facilities, by Source, Fiscal Years 2013 through 2018.

While third-party collections at federally operated IHS facilities collectively increased from fiscal year 2013 through 2018, there was significant variation in changes for individual facilities. IHS officials we

[26] According to our analysis of IHS coverage data, the number of patients seeking care at federally operated IHS facilities changed less than one-half of one percent between fiscal years 2013 and 2018.

interviewed noted several reasons why third-party collections may vary over time and by location, including

- the size of the facility and any changes in the number of providers, patients, or business office staff that process billing and collections;
- the ability to collect payment from certain tribal health insurance, which may opt to not pay for services provided to enrolled members; and
- the number of patients enrolled in Medicaid managed care plans, which may identify IHS facilities as out-of-network providers and not pay for covered services.[27]

IHS and federally operated facility officials we interviewed noted that gains in health insurance coverage during this time period contributed to increases in collections. In addition, officials we interviewed from most of the 12 area offices and 11 selected federally operated IHS facilities described steps they took to enhance collections. More specifically, officials from seven area offices discussed initiating steps to improve billing and collections functions for federally operated IHS facilities in their area; at one area office this involved creating a new area-level position focused on revenue enhancement at federally operated IHS facilities. Additionally, officials we interviewed at six federally operated IHS facilities identified steps they took to enhance the accuracy and efficiency of facilities' collections, noting efforts such as improving training related to coding and billing. For example, officials at one of these facilities described convening a team to review why all claims related to a specific service were being rejected. The team then instituted changes to

[27] According to officials from one federally operated facility, while the state Medicaid program was supposed to enroll tribal members in a fee-for-service plan that would enable enrollees to use such coverage at their facility, some tribal members had been erroneously enrolled in a Medicaid managed care plan, making it difficult for the facility to collect payment for covered services. Officials from a few tribally operated facilities and area Indian health boards also reported similar challenges.

their billing procedures that resulted in the facility collecting payments for these services.

Officials from Selected Tribally Operated Facilities and Tribal Organizations Described Increases in Health Insurance Coverage and Third-Party Collections at Some Tribal Facilities

Officials we interviewed at selected tribally operated facilities and tribal organizations—including national tribal organizations and area Indian health boards—described increases in health insurance coverage and collections at some tribally operated facilities that occurred from 2013 through 2018. Specifically, some tribal organization officials reported increases in coverage at facilities located in states that had expanded their Medicaid programs, compared with those that had not. For example, officials at one tribally operated facility noted that the percent of their patients with health coverage increased by 10 percentage points from 2013 to 2018. Similar to federally operated IHS facilities, officials we interviewed from some tribally operated facilities said they focused on screening patients for coverage at the time of service, including by increasing the number of patient benefits coordinators and always having staff available to help enroll patients in coverage. These officials also noted that they conducted outreach and enrollment activities to inform patients of the importance of having coverage and benefitting from outreach and education activities conducted directly by local tribes, including through messages that emphasized the importance of coverage for the tribe and tribally operated facility. Officials from a national tribal organization told us that one tribally operated facility placed stickers on all equipment purchased with third-party collections as a way to educate patients about the benefits of having health insurance coverage and to encourage further enrollment in coverage. Officials we interviewed at selected tribally operated facilities and national tribal organizations also described increases in third-party collections that occurred from 2013 through 2018 at many tribally operated facilities— particularly those located in Medicaid expansion states. For example, officials from one tribally operated facility told us that they anticipated that their third-party collections for 2018 would be more than twice the amount they collected for 2013.[28] Similar to federally operated IHS facilities, officials we interviewed from some tribally operated facilities noted that their facilities had enhanced collections by making improvements to their billing processes and taking steps to increase patient volume. For example, officials at one tribally operated facility said they recently began allowing non-tribal members to receive care at their facility—an option available to tribally operated facilities but not to federally operated IHS facilities—as a way to increase third-party collections and bolster the facility's long-term sustainability.[29]

Some officials also noted that not all tribally operated facilities experienced increases in collections, in part because of decreases or limitations in the number of providers, patients, or business office staff that process billing and collections. Similar to federally operated IHS facilities, officials from tribally operated facilities noted that the enrollment of patients in Medicaid managed care plans also reduced their ability to collect payment for covered services because these plans often identify the facilities as out-of-network providers and therefore do not pay for covered services provided onsite.

INCREASES IN COVERAGE AND COLLECTIONS REPORTEDLY HELPED SELECTED FEDERALLY OPERATED AND TRIBALLY OPERATED FACILITIES TO CONTINUE OPERATIONS AND EXPAND SERVICES

Officials we interviewed from selected federally operated and tribally operated facilities stated that increases in coverage and third-party

[28] Final 2018 collections amounts for this facility were unavailable at the time of our interview.

[29] Federally operated IHS facilities generally provide services to eligible AI/AN and certain non-Indians, such as children of eligible AI/AN. See 25 U.S.C. § 1680c; 42 C.F.R. §§ 136.12, 136.14 (2018). Tribally operated facilities, however, have in some cases chosen to provide services to a broader patient population.

collections helped them to (1) continue their facilities' operations, (2) expand the services they offer onsite at their facilities, and (3) expand the services they cover offsite through IHS's PRC program.

Continued Operations

Officials we interviewed from all 17 selected federally operated and tribally operated facilities noted that they used increased third-party collections to fund their continued operations. Even as officials we interviewed from nearly all of the 11 selected federally operated IHS facilities reported that their facilities' third-party collections had grown from fiscal years 2013 to 2018, officials from most of these facilities also said they relied more heavily on these collections to support their continued operations. Officials we interviewed from all of the IHS area offices told us that third-party collections provide a vital source of funding for federally operated IHS facilities in their area. These collections allowed them to maintain a level of operations that would otherwise be challenging, for reasons such as increasing costs of payroll and of maintaining an aging infrastructure. In addition, officials we interviewed from most of the selected federally operated IHS facilities reported using third-party collections to fund a substantial and increasing portion of their payroll costs. Officials at many of the IHS area offices and most of the selected federally operated IHS facilities we interviewed also reported using third-party collections to ensure that their facility met all required standards, including those required for ongoing accreditation, or to undertake any needed maintenance such as by repairing roofs and heating systems. Some of these officials also reported using third-party collections to repair or replace medical equipment that was broken or had exceeded its intended lifespan. Table 2 displays examples of how selected federally operated and tribally operated facilities reported using third-party collections.

Table 2. Examples of How Selected Federally Operated and Tribally Operated Facilities Used Third-Party Collections to Continue Operations or Expand Services, Fiscal Years 2013 through 2018

Category	Examples
Providers	• Hiring or contracting to offer increased onsite services through primary care physicians, nurse practitioners, behavioral health specialists, cardiologists, dentists, podiatrists, and others. • Offering more competitive wages to assist with recruiting providers. • Offering recruitment, relocation, and retention bonuses for providers. • Funding efforts to construct and make available government housing for providers near facilities. • Developing a training program for local tribal members to become health care providers.
Medical equipment	• Repairing, purchasing, or contracting to provide enhanced access to diagnostic medical equipment including ultrasound, x-ray, computed tomography scan, and magnetic resonance imaging machines. • Purchasing hospital beds and stretchers, dental equipment and chairs, surgical devices, electrocardiogram machines, and patient monitoring systems.
Health promotion and education activities	• Continuing to provide intensive diabetes case management interventions to reduce cardiovascular disease after expiration of IHS's Healthy Hearts grant funding. • Establishing or continuing diabetes education and nutrition programs. • Providing a free anticoagulation clinic. • Establishing targeted interventions to reduce the number of patients with uncontrolled high blood pressure.
Expanding and renovating facilities	• Repairing facility infrastructure, including roofs and heating systems. • Renovating existing space, such as operating rooms, emergency rooms, and patient care areas to improve patient flow and meet industry standards. • Expanding a facility by adding exam rooms within the current facility or constructing a new building to be part of an existing facility. • Purchasing modular buildings or leasing space to increase capacity. • Enhancing existing information technology infrastructure, including by implementing an electronic health records system and replacing wiring and servers.
Purchased/Referred Care (PRC)a	• Supplementing appropriated funds for PRC to enhance access to offsite services.

Source: Indian Health Service. | GAO-19-612.

Note: Table reflects information gathered through interviews with officials from 12 Indian Health Service area offices and 17 selected federally operated and tribally operated facilities.

[a]PRC programs enable patients to obtain health care services from private providers if the patients meet certain requirements and funding is available.

Expanded Services Onsite

Officials we interviewed from most of the 17 selected federally operated and tribally operated facilities told us they used increased third-party collections to expand the volume or scope of services they offered onsite as a way to better meet patients' medical needs.[30] With respect to increasing the volume of services provided, officials at most of these facilities said they added providers and medical equipment to provide patients with more timely access to services. In one example, officials from a federally operated IHS hospital said they added about 30 additional nurses from 2013 to 2018 as a result of increased third-party collections. As a result of increases in the number of providers at their facilities, officials we interviewed from several federally operated IHS facilities said they were able to schedule appointments for patients more quickly, which reduced wait times for an appointment—including two facilities that reported being able to newly offer same-day appointments.[31] Officials from facilities that expanded the scope of services provided said they did so by adding new specialties, such as behavioral health and dentistry, purchasing new medical equipment such as hospital beds, dental chairs, and magnetic resonance imaging machines, and funding health promotion and education activities such as those related to diabetes education. (See Figure 6).

To support efforts to expand services and bolster their sustainability, officials from most of the 17 federally operated and tribally operated facilities said they used third-party collections to offer more competitive salaries and bonuses for providers. In addition, officials from a few of the 12 IHS area offices told us that federally operated facilities in their area used third-party collections to fund projects to construct nearby housing for

---

[30] While officials from most of the selected facilities reported adding services that could be reimbursed through third-party collections to help keep those services sustainable, officials from a few federally operated IHS facilities also noted they added services such as acupuncture and chiropractor services that are not traditionally reimbursed through insurance as a way to further meet the needs of their patient populations.

[31] We previously reported that a lack of primary care providers, as well as aging infrastructure and equipment, were significant obstacles to IHS in ensuring that patients receive timely care. See GAO, *Indian Health Service: Actions Needed to Ensure Patients' Access to Timely Care,* GAO-16-333 (Washington, D.C.: Mar. 29, 2016).

providers.[32] In another example, officials from a national tribal organization noted that the use of third-party collections to enhance provider salaries at one facility led to a decrease in provider turnover from about 40 percent prior to 2014 to 14 percent in 2018. In addition, officials from many of the IHS area offices told us that some federally operated facilities in their area reported using third-party collections accumulated over multiple years to make investments in expanding their facilities to provide the space necessary to support these additional services. For example, according to IHS officials,

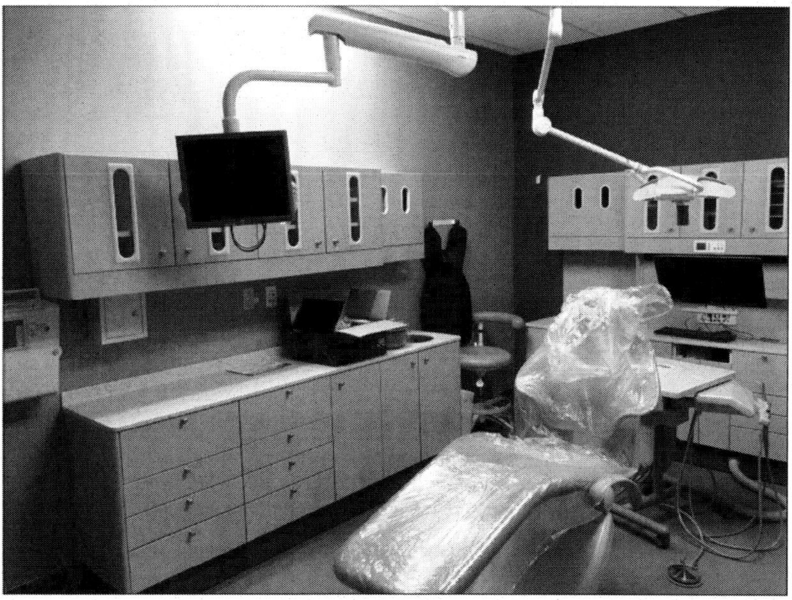

This dental chair with x-ray capability allows dentists to view x-rays while performing oral surgery.

Source: GAO. | GAO-19-612.

Figure 6. Example of Equipment Purchased with Third-Party Collections at a Federally Operated Indian Health Service (IHS) Facility.

---

[32] In 2018, we reported that the overall vacancy rate for IHS providers was 25 percent, and we identified challenges the agency faces with respect to recruiting and retaining providers, including difficulties matching local market salaries. See GAO, *Indian Health Service: Agency Faces Ongoing Challenges Filling Provider Vacancies*, GAO-18-580 (Washington, D.C.: Aug.15, 2018).

- one federally operated IHS facility reported using $7 million in third-party collections to fund an over 11,000 square foot expansion to house an expanded emergency room and a new urgent care clinic;
- two federally operated IHS facilities reported using third-party collections to purchase modular buildings to provide medical services such as audiology, behavioral health, and dental services; and
- one federally operated IHS facility reported saving third-party collections for six years to fund the construction of a new 23,000 square foot building to provide additional space for an increased volume of services, including dental, optometry and physical therapy services, and to pay for the new medical equipment to support these services (see Figure 7).

Officials from some IHS area offices stated that the extent to which federally operated IHS facilities in their area invested in expanding onsite services largely depended on the level of facilities' third-party collections. Specifically, facilities experiencing larger increases in collections, such as larger facilities or those located in Medicaid expansion states, were able to invest more heavily in an expansion of onsite services compared to those that had lower increases in collections, according to these officials.

To identify their facilities' needs, officials from federally operated and tribally operated facilities reported using a variety of approaches. For example, officials from three IHS area offices and one tribally operated facility said they analyzed PRC data to identify the services that patients were obtaining through that program, and worked to bring those services onsite. Officials from two federally operated IHS facilities also noted that they incorporated local tribal input as they identified local needs and projects to fund.[33] For example, these officials told us that their facilities

[33] Federal agencies are required in certain circumstances to consult with tribes on infrastructure projects and other activities that may affect tribal natural and cultural resources. We recently examined key factors tribes and selected federal agencies identified that hinder effective consultation on infrastructure projects and steps agencies have taken to facilitate

were in the process of adding new specialty services onsite, including acupuncture, chiropractor, and eye clinic services, at the request of their local tribes.

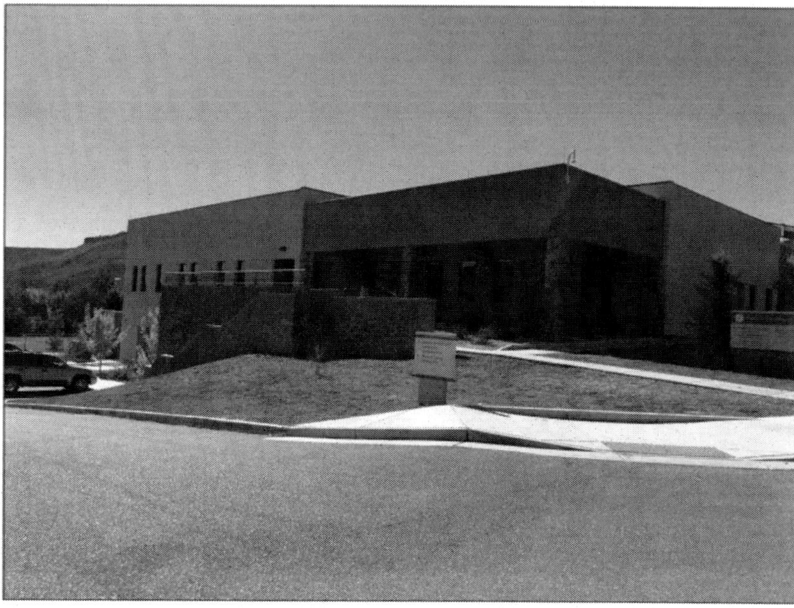

An HIS hospital used third-party collections saved over a 6-year period to finance the construction of new space that served to expand an existing facility by increasing the space available for existing programs and services, including dental, optometry, and physical therapy services.

Source: GAO. | GAO-19-612.

Figure 7. Example of a Federally Operated Indian Health Service (IHS) Facility Expansion Funded With Third-Party Collections.

The recent growth in third-party collections has made it possible for many federally operated IHS facilities to consider funding a range of projects, and IHS officials said they relied on established procedures to fund these projects. According to IHS officials, local facility officials draft annual spending proposals to identify the resources, including third-party collections, that they would like to use to address their facilities' needs.

tribal consultation. See GAO, *Tribal Consultation: Additional Federal Actions Needed for Infrastructure Projects,* GAO-19-22 (Washington, D.C.: Mar. 20, 2019).

These proposals are provided to each facility's governing board for review; the governing board is comprised of area office and facility officials whose top priority is maintaining accreditation and ensuring patient safety at each facility, according to IHS officials. Once these basic needs are met, IHS officials told us that facilities may begin to identify and fund projects to expand access to health services.

Expanding Services Offsite

Officials from IHS, as well as some of the 17 selected federally operated and tribally operated facilities, told us that increased coverage and collections allowed for an expansion in the complexity of services provided offsite through the PRC program. Specifically, officials reported that an increase in the percent of patients with health insurance, coupled with facilities' enhanced onsite services, has led PRC programs to be able to expand the level of care that they can offer. For example, they stated that increases in the health insurance coverage of patients have led to a smaller percent of patients needing to access PRC, since patients may use their coverage to obtain needed services directly from other private providers. In addition, an expansion of available services onsite at federally operated and tribally operated facilities resulting from increased collections reduced the need for some patients to use PRC.[34]

From 2013 through 2018, most IHS-administered PRC programs moved from covering only the most acute and emergent cases to funding nearly all types of care covered through the PRC program, according to our analysis of IHS data and interviews with agency officials.

---

[34] Officials we interviewed also noted several other factors that affected their ability to expand services offsite. For example, IHS officials reported that beginning in 2016, they were able to use lower Medicare-like rates to pay for outpatient PRC services, which helped them to extend PRC resources. In addition, officials from a few IHS area offices told us that some federally operated IHS facilities in their area had supplemented their PRC funding with third-party collections, including at the request of a local tribe, in order to further enhance their ability to fund offsite patient services.

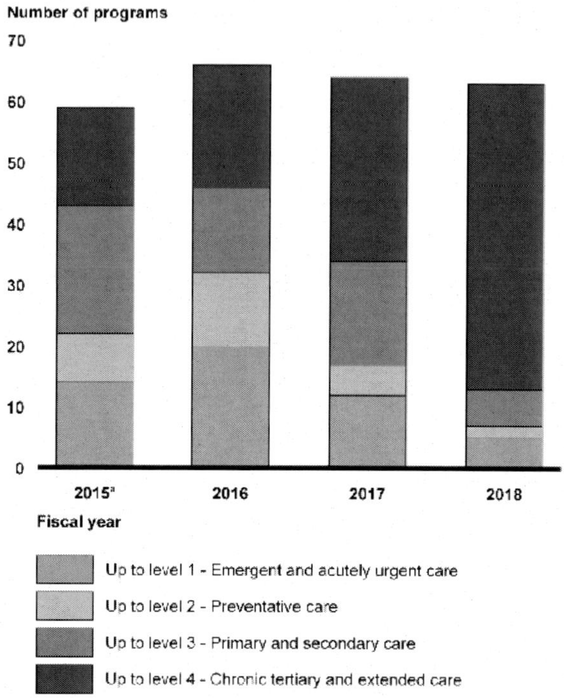

Source: GAO analysis of Indian Health Service (IHS) data. | GAO-19-612.

Notes: PRC programs enable patients to obtain health care services from private providers if the patients meet certain requirements and funding is available. IHS-administered PRC programs follow the agency's medical priority system for the use of funds. These programs first pay for all of the highest priority services—for example, priority 1, and then all or some of the lower priority services—depending on the availability of funds. Programs funding services at levels 2, 3, or 4 therefore must also fund all services at higher priority levels. IHS priority level 5 refers to services excluded from PRC, which include cosmetic and experimental procedures. Tribes may opt to administer PRC programs but are not required to use the IHS medical priority system. The number of HIS administered PRC programs differs for each year because of changes in tribal administration of the programs. According to an IHS official, in fiscal year 2018, 39 percent of PRC appropriations were administered by IHS; the remaining 61 percent were administered by tribes.

[a]Two IHS-administered PRC programs did not provide data for 2015.

Figure 8. Medical Priority Levels Funded through Purchased/Referred Care (PRC) Programs Administered by IHS, Fiscal Years 2015 through 2018.

Specifically, IHS officials we interviewed told us that prior to 2014, most PRC programs administered by the agency were only able to fund care for the most acute and emergent cases—referred to as priority level 1. Our analysis of IHS data showed that these PRC programs were increasingly able to fund additional medical priority levels of care each year from fiscal year 2015— the first year that such data were available—through fiscal year 2018, with most IHS-administered programs funding care through priority level 4 in fiscal year 2018. (See Figure 8).

Officials we interviewed at some of the 17 selected federally operated and tribally operated facilities that had been able to both expand services onsite and offsite through PRC funds told us that these changes have made a large impact on patients' health and quality of life. For example, officials at some federally operated IHS facilities reported that having more providers onsite has allowed them to offer patients more rapid access to care, and officials from some tribally operated facilities reported that an expansion of onsite services has allowed them to serve more patients. Officials at some of the selected federally operated and tribally operated facilities reported that an expansion of onsite services has also reduced the need for some patients to travel long distances to obtain diagnostic services and specialty care through the PRC program. In addition, officials from two IHS area offices noted that PRC has been able to pay for services such as patients' long-awaited knee and hip replacements, which have enabled patients to return to normal activities of life and reduce their need for pain management.

AGENCY COMMENTS

We provided a draft of this chapter for review and comment to the Secretary of Health and Human Services. The Department did not have any comments on the draft report.

As agreed with your offices, unless you publicly announce the contents of this chapter earlier, we plan no further distribution until 30 days from the report date. At that time, we will send copies to the Secretary of the Department of Health and Human Services and other interested parties.

Jessica Farb
Director, Health Care.

APPENDIX I: ESTIMATED HEALTH INSURANCE COVERAGE OF THE AMERICAN INDIAN AND ALASKA NATIVE POPULATION, 2013 THROUGH 2017

In the years since the Patient Protection and Affordable Care Act (PPACA) authorized states to expand access to Medicaid and offer health insurance through the exchanges in 2014, the percent of American Indian and Alaska Native (AI/AN) in the general population with health insurance has increased. Specifically, according to an analysis of U.S. Census Bureau's American Community Survey data, the percent of nonelderly AI/ANs with health insurance coverage increased from 70 percent in 2013 to 78 percent in 2017.[35] (See Figure 9).

While the estimated percent of AI/AN nationwide reporting health insurance coverage increased from 2013 to 2017, these increases in coverage were not evenly distributed among the states, according to an analysis of U.S. Census Bureau's American Community Survey data.[36]

---

[35] Kaiser Family Foundation, *Changes in Health Coverage by Race and Ethnicity since Implementation of the ACA, 2013-2017* (San Francisco, Calif.: Feb. 13, 2019).

[36] Kaiser Family Foundation, *Health and Health Care for American Indians and Alaskan Natives (AIANs) in the United States* (San Francisco, Calif.: May 10, 2019).

The estimated percent of AI/AN reporting health insurance increased more in states that expanded Medicaid compared to those that did not. (See Figure 10).

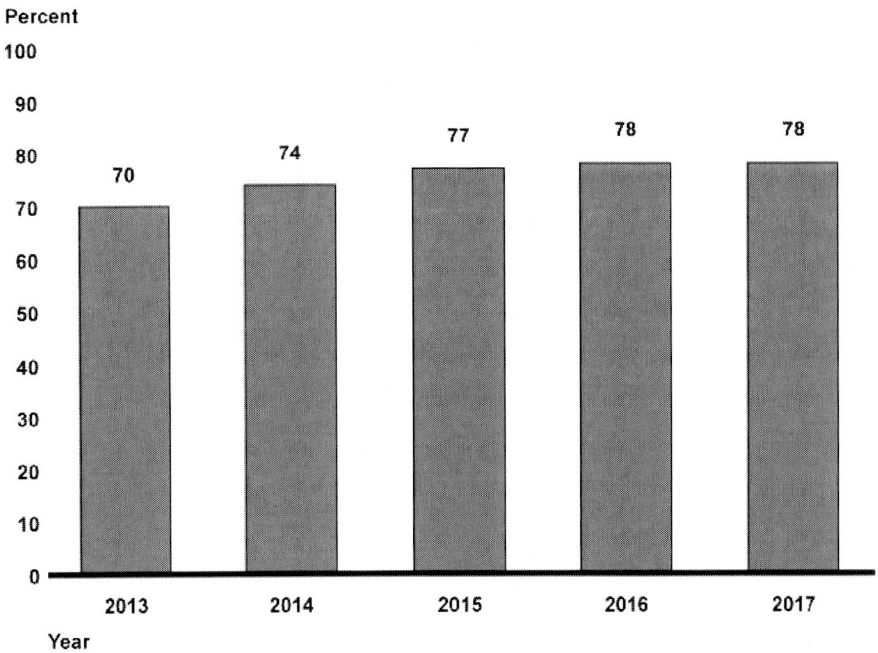

Source: Kaiser Family Foundation analysis of U.S. Census Bureau's American Community Survey data. | GAO-19-612.

Note: Data include nonelderly individuals aged 0 to 64 who self-identified as non-Hispanic American Indians and Alaska Natives.

Figure 9. Estimated Health Insurance Coverage of the Nonelderly American Indian and Alaska Native Population, 2013 through 2017.

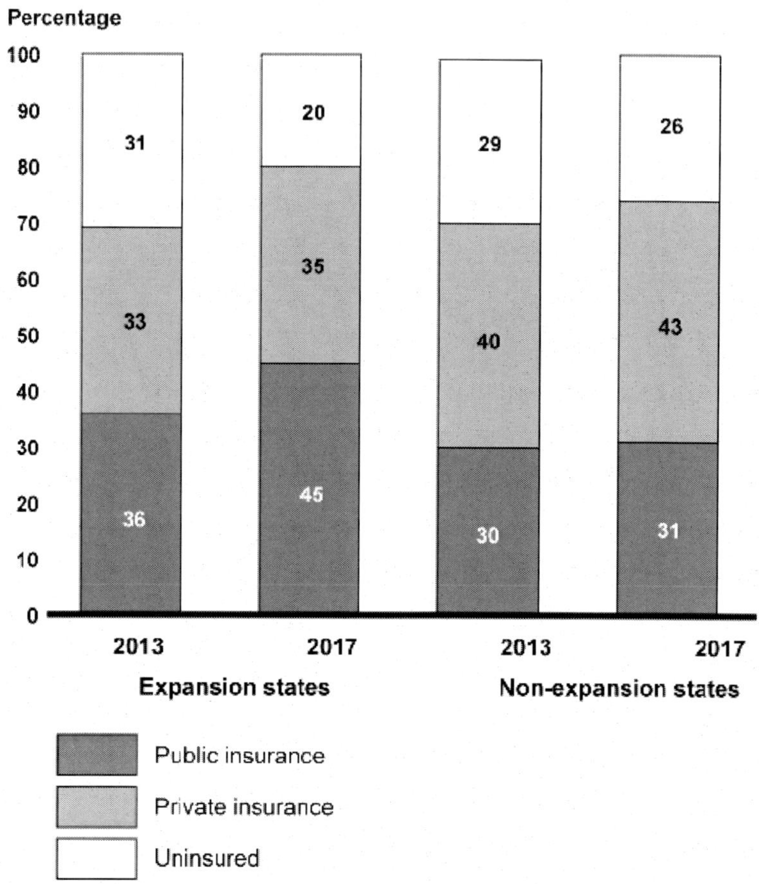

Source: Kaiser Family Foundation analysis of U.S. Census Bureau's American Community Survey data. | GAO-19-612.

Note: Data include nonelderly individuals aged 0 to 64 who self-identified as American Indians and Alaska Natives and excludes those identified as Hispanic or of mixed races.

Figure 10. Estimated Health Insurance Coverage among Nonelderly American Indian and Alaska Natives, 2013 and 2017, by State Medicaid Expansion Status.

INDEX

A

B

C

D

E

F

G

H

I

L

M

N

O

P

R

S